PANCE FLASHCARDS
PHYSICIAN ASSISTANT NATIONAL CERTIFYING EXAM

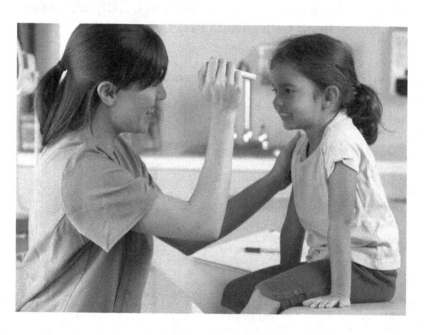

Doris A. Rapp, PharmD, PA-C
University of Kentucky
Lexington, KY

Research & Education Association
Visit our website at: www.rea.com

Research & Education Association
61 Ethel Road West
Piscataway, New Jersey 08854
E-mail: info@rea.com

**PANCE (Physician Assistant National Certifying Exam)
Flashcard Book with Online Practice**

Printed in the United States of America

ISBN-13: 978-0-7386-1176-1
ISBN-10: 0-7386-1176-X

Cover image © Catherine Yeulet/iStock/Thinkstock

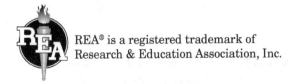

About this Book + Online Practice

If you have completed an accredited Physician Assistant educational program and are getting ready to take the Physician Assistant National Certifying Exam, our PANCE prep package will help make sure you're prepared.

Derived from the National Commission on Certification of Physician Assistants' content blueprint for the PANCE, our flashcards and quizzes cover dermatology, EENT, cardiovascular, neurology, pulmonary, and more.

Start your prep by studying the book's 400 flashcards which include basic and detailed information regarding diseases, diagnosis, and management, important facts and details, as well as patient scenarios seen in clinical practice.

Then, go to the online REA Study Center (*www.rea.com/studycenter*) to see how well you've mastered the material by testing yourself with our 4 online quizzes. These 10-question quizzes feature automatic scoring with diagnostic feedback that identifies any areas in need of further review, helping to ensure that you are ready for test day.

Also at the REA Study Center, you'll find seven invaluable medical reference charts that you can return to time and again:

- Anatomy I
- Anatomy II
- Medical Abbreviations
- Medical Terms: The Basics
- Medical Terms: The Body
- Muscular System
- Skeletal System

These charts provide quick, easy access to important facts you need to know and are great for last-minute review.

Good luck on the exam!

About Our Author

Doris A. Rapp, PharmD, PA-C received her B.S. in Biology from Tennessee Technological University and her B.S. in Pharmacy from the University of Kentucky College of Pharmacy, Lexington, Kentucky. Dr. Rapp then went on to earn her Certificate in Physician Assistant Studies from the University of Kentucky College of Allied Health and her PharmD from the University of Kentucky College of Pharmacy. She is currently the Division Director of the Physician Assistant Studies Program at the University of Kentucky.

About Research & Education Association

Founded in 1959, Research & Education Association (REA) is dedicated to publishing the finest and most effective educational materials—including study guides and test preps—for students in middle school, high school, college, graduate school, and beyond. Today, REA's wide-ranging catalog is a leading resource for teachers, students, and professionals. Visit *www.rea.com* to see a complete listing of all our titles.

Acknowledgments

We would like to thank Larry B. Kling, Vice President, Editorial, for his overall direction; Pam Weston, Publisher, for setting the quality standards for production integrity and managing the publication to completion; John Cording, Vice President, Technology, for coordinating the design and development of the REA Study Center; Kelli Wilkins, Managing Editor, for project management; and Claudia Petrilli, Graphic Designer, for prepress production and for designing our cover. In addition, we extend our thanks to S4 Carlisle for technically reviewing the manuscript and to Lisa Naser, MS, PA-C for writing the online quizzes.

Questions

Women's Health/Reproductive

A 34-year-old woman requests a combination oral contraceptive for birth control. Which one of the following would be a contraindication to prescribing oral contraceptives for this patient?

(A)   A history of controlled hypertension
(B)   A family history of ovarian cancer
(C)   A history of thromboembolic disease
(D)   A current history of smoking

Your Answer _____

_____

Women's Health/Reproductive

A recently married 28-year-old female presents with uncomplicated cystitis. She is otherwise healthy. She currently uses barrier birth control methods but has plans to discontinue this soon, as she wants to become pregnant. Which of the following supplemental vitamins or minerals would you advise this patient to begin taking?

(A)   Ferrous sulfate
(B)   Calcium carbonate
(C)   Ascorbic acid
(D)   Folic acid

Your Answer _____

_____

Correct Answers

A–1

(C) Oral contraceptives have been associated with an increased risk of developing blood clots (thromboembolic disease) by as much as a fourfold increase. Currently available oral contraceptives (OCs) contain low doses of estrogen and do not carry the contraindications of earlier, larger doses of OCs. However, one should maintain close supervision of women who have controlled hypertension, are current smokers, have a family history of ovarian cancer, and are prescribed oral contraceptives.

A–2

(D) When planning for a pregnancy, folic acid supplementation of 400 micrograms daily beginning 3 months prior to conception is recommended to decrease the likelihood of neural tube defects in the baby. Once pregnancy is established, the mother-to-be should be prescribed a prenatal vitamin supplement to help meet the required demands of pregnancy and to assure that a steady supply of nutrients reaches the developing fetus.

Questions

Dermatology

A patient presents with a skin lesion that he describes as painless when he first noticed it, but now, about 3–4 hours later, he describes the lesion as quite painful. Physical examination reveals a ring of pallor immediately around the lesion (bleb), with a surrounding area of erythema. Your initial impression is

(A) erythema nodosum
(B) brown recluse spider bite
(C) toxic epidermal necrolysis
(D) allergic dermatitis

Your Answer _____

_____

EENT

A 68-year-old female presents to your practice with complaints of tinnitus and a declining ability to understand speech if spoken too quickly or when background noise is present. An in-office otoscopic exam revealed no visible abnormalities. You suspect this elderly woman is suffering from

(A) presbycusis
(B) cerumen impaction
(C) otosclerosis
(D) presbyopia

Your Answer _____

_____

Correct Answers

A–3

(B) Brown recluse spider venom produces both localized and systemic effects. Early symptoms include pain that develops between 2 and 10 hours after the initial bite. Soon thereafter, a ring of pallor, secondary to vasoconstriction, surrounds the bite. Beyond the pallor, the skin is erythematous. The bleb, at the center, becomes necrotic after a few days. Erythema nodosum can be due to a variety of causes and presents as tender, erythematous nodules usually seen on the shins. Toxic epidermal necrolysis is a widespread, life-threatening skin condition that frequently results from a reaction to medications. Allergic dermatitis presents as an itchy skin condition and its cause can be traced to an allergy to a specific agent or group of agents.

A–4

(A) Presbycusis is a common auditory disorder in which there is bilateral sensorineural hearing loss associated with aging. It is caused by degenerative changes in the inner ear and auditory nerves. Cerumen impaction causes a blockage of the external ear canal and may cause symptoms of partial hearing loss, itching and tinnitus, along with a feeling of fullness in the ear. A diagnosis can be made by otoscopic examination of the ear. Otosclerosis is a hereditary condition usually noticed between the late teens and 30 years of age. It causes a progressive conductive hearing loss, typically of low-to-medium pitch sounds. Presbyopia describes the inability of the eyes to focus on near objects as one ages.

Questions

Cardiovascular

From the following list, which symptoms are most likely to be present in a patient with heart failure?

    a. Shortness of breath while lying in bed
    b. Pain in the left arm
    c. Epigastric pain
    d. Cough, especially at night
    e. Shortness of breath on exertion

(A) a and c
(B) a, b, and c
(C) b and d
(D) a, d, and e

Your Answer _____

_____

Correct Answers

(D) A person with heart failure has a cardiac disorder that impairs the ability of the ventricle(s) to function as a pump, i.e., to fill with or eject blood to meet the needs of the body. This results in a variety of signs and symptoms primarily manifested as fluid retention with subsequent shortness of breath (a and e), fatigue, and decreased exercise tolerance. Because of fluid retention in the lungs, the patient may develop a cough that worsens when the patient is supine due to the fluid shift, such as at night (d). Pain in the left arm and epigastric pain are more commonly associated with myocardial infarction.

Questions

Neurology

Mr. Brown, age 59, is brought to the emergency department and the triage nurse suspects he has had a stroke.
The family states that Mr. Brown appeared normal until
about 2 hours ago when he began to have slurred speech
and wanted to lie down. Mr. Brown is now comatose. His
B/P is 160/90 mm Hg; blood glucose 110 mg/dL; and ECG
is WNL. Initial treatment for this patient is

(A) clopidogrel
(B) intravenous heparin
(C) intravenous rt-PA
(D) aspirin

Your Answer _____

_____

Correct Answers

A–6

(C) This patient meets all the inclusion criteria for administration of rt-PA and, after consent from the family, should be given a dose of 0.9 mg/kg (maximum of 90 mg) infused over one hour, with 10% of the total dose infused over the first minute. Aspirin is recommended for most acute stroke patients, however, it should be withheld for at least 24 hours after administration of thrombolytics. Clopidogrel may be used in patients allergic to aspirin, although its beneficial effects are unproven. Studies have demonstrated that IV heparin offers no appreciable benefit for most patients and should not be administered within 24 hours of thrombolytic therapy.

Questions

Cardiovascular

The pain of chronic peripheral arterial disease, manifesting as intermittent claudication, has which of the following characteristics?

(A) It is associated with swelling of the affected extremity.
(B) It is increased with exercise.
(C) It is associated with a dilated saphenous system on the affected side.
(D) The patient will have a positive Homan's sign.

Your Answer _____

_____

Cardiovascular

A 50-year-old male presents to the emergency department with a suspected myocardial infarction. Examinations helpful in making the diagnosis *at the time of his arrival* would be

(A) electrocardiogram
(B) chest X-ray
(C) elevated CK and CK-MB enzymes
(D) elevated myoglobin

Your Answer _____

_____

Correct Answers

A–7

(B) Peripheral arterial disease is characterized by pain that develops with exercise and is relieved by rest. Swelling is more often present in venous insufficiency and may be evident by dilated saphenous veins. A positive Homan's sign is indicative of venous thrombosis even though a patient may have a thrombus and not have a positive Homan's sign.

A–8

(A) All of the procedures would be obtained on a patient suspected of having a myocardial infarction, along with the cardiac specific marker for acute MI, troponin. Of the choices presented in the question, the ECG will give the most rapid information, although a patient may be having an MI and have a normal ECG. CK and CK-MB enzymes rise after an MI but the rise is usually delayed for 3–4 hours. Also, myoglobin will rise in a person with an infarcted myocardium but it is nonspecific, being found also in skeletal muscle.

Questions

Women's Health/Reproductive

Which of the following combinations accurately describes the normal progression of labor?

(A) Stage I usually lasts no longer than 6–8 hours and is characterized by Braxton-Hicks contractions.

(B) Stage II is active labor lasting from 4–6 hours. The cervix is dilated to approximately 8 cm and contractions are 3–5 minutes apart.

(C) Stage III lasts 15 minutes to 1.5 hours. The cervix dilates to 10 cm and contractions are 60 to 90 seconds long and 2–3 minutes apart. Delivery is expected soon.

(D) None of the above statements are true.

Your Answer _____

_____

Correct Answers

(D) Braxton-Hicks contractions that are perceived by the patient occur late in pregnancy but are not associated with dilation of the cervix. Stage I is the interval between the onset of labor and full cervical dilation (10 cm). Stage II encompasses complete cervical dilation with delivery of the baby. Stage III begins immediately after delivery of the baby and ends with delivery of the placenta. The final stage is Stage IV which is the immediate postpartum period of approximately 1 to 4 hours after delivery of the placenta.

Questions

Cardiovascular

A 32-year-old white male presents for an insurance physical. He is asymptomatic and denies significant past medical history. His physical examination is essentially normal except that he has a blood pressure of 140/90 mm Hg in both arms. What is the most appropriate intervention at this time?

(A) No diagnosis: Return in 2 weeks to recheck the blood pressure.

(B) No diagnosis: Obtain an electrocardiogram, complete metabolic panel, and urinalysis and return in 2 weeks to recheck the blood pressure.

(C) Stage I primary hypertension: Obtain labs mentioned in (B) above and begin nonpharmacologic therapy.

(D) Stage I primary hypertension: Obtain labs mentioned in (B) above and begin pharmacologic therapy.

Your Answer _____

_____

Correct Answers

A–10

(A) This appears to be a healthy 32-year-old gentleman according to the history. He should not be classified as hypertensive unless he has a proven sustained elevation of his blood pressure. It would be appropriate to instruct the patient to measure his blood pressure at home daily (or twice daily), keep a record of the readings, and return for an office visit in two weeks. The JNC-7 report classifies a well-documented sustained blood pressure of 140/90 as Stage I hypertension and recommends initiation of pharmacologic therapy along with lifestyle modifications.

Questions

Cardiovascular

Which antihypertensive agent would be most preferred in a patient with coexisting diabetes mellitus?

(A) Thiazide diuretic
(B) Calcium channel blocker
(C) Beta adrenergic blocker
(D) ACE inhibitor

Your Answer _____

_____

Pulmonary

Which process most accurately reflects the current understanding of the pathogenesis of asthma?

(A) Chronic airway inflammation
(B) Activated macrophage release of leukotrienes and tumor necrosis factor alpha
(C) Inhalation of dust
(D) An imbalance between protease and antiprotease activities in the lungs

Your Answer _____

_____

Correct Answers

A–11

(D) Placebo controlled trials in diabetic patients have shown the efficacy of ACE inhibitors, diuretics, and beta blockers as initial therapy in lowering blood pressure. However, ACE inhibitors have also been shown to slow progression of diabetic nephropathy, making this the best first line choice. Studies have also shown that the use of ACE inhibitors in high risk hypertensive patients slows the occurrence of cardiovascular events, i.e., stroke, coronary artery disease, etc.

A–12

(A) Asthma is defined as a chronic inflammatory disorder of the airways. Choices (B) and (C) are more pathogenic of emphysema, and pneumoconiosis results from inhalation of various kinds of dust particles. Imbalances between protease and antiprotease activity is being studied as a cause for alveolar wall destruction.

Questions

Pulmonary

Bronchial breathing, egophony, whispered pectoriloquy, diminished fremitus, and dullness to percussion are most consistent with which diagnosis?

(A) Pneumothorax
(B) Upper lobe atelectasis
(C) Consolidated pneumonia
(D) Pleural effusion

Your Answer _____

Women's Health

Which diagnosis must ALWAYS be excluded in a female patient with an acute abdomen?

(A) Ectopic pregnancy
(B) Ovarian cyst
(C) Endometriosis
(D) Appendicitis

Your Answer _____

Correct Answers

A-13

(B) The findings are consistent with upper lobe atelectasis. If it were lower lobe atelectasis, the patient would have diminished or absent breath sounds. Pneumothorax presents with diminished to absent breath sounds, diminished or absent whispered voice sounds, and hyperresonance to percussion. It usually occurs in one lung only. Consolidated pneumonia presents with a variety of crackles and/or rhonchi along with bronchial breath sounds, egophony, whispered pectoriloquy, and increased fremitus in the area of consolidation. Pleural effusion presents with diminished or absent breath sounds, bronchophony, whispered pectoriloquy, an occasional friction rub, and dullness to percussion.

A-14

(A) Ectopic pregnancy (implantation outside the uterine cavity) is incompatible with continuing the pregnancy and carries the risk of catastrophic bleeding if it erodes into blood vessels or ruptures through the fallopian tube. Ovarian cysts usually resolve spontaneously or may be managed by pharmacological agents. Endometriosis causes a wide variation in symptoms with pelvic pain being the most common finding. It is not usually associated with an acute abdomen. Acute appendicitis typically produces pain in the right lower quadrant of the abdomen and is a cause of an acute abdomen. In the female of childbearing potential, however, the best answer to the question is selection (A).

Questions

Respiratory

The most common pathogen causing community acquired pneumonia (CAP) is

(A) *Streptococcus pneumoniae*
(B) *Mycoplasma pneumoniae*
(C) *Hemophilus influenza*
(D) *Klebsiella pneumoniae*

Your Answer _____

_____

Gastrointestinal

The diagnosis of appendicitis is MOST likely to be missed in which age group?

(A) 1–6 years
(B) 11–20 years
(C) Over 65 years
(D) Both (A) and (C) are correct.

Your Answer _____

_____

Correct Answers

A–15

(A) *Streptococcus pneumoniae* causes 20–50% of the cases of CAP; *Mycoplasma pneumoniae* is responsible for 10–30%; *Hemophilus influenza* 5–10%; and *Klebsiella pneumoniea* 1–3% of the cases.

A–16

(D) Young children have difficulty in expressing their symptoms clearly and elderly patients may have a reduced inflammatory reaction, making diagnosis more difficult in these age groups. Appendicitis reaches its peak between the ages of 10 and 20, and approximately 80% of cases occur before the age of 45.

Questions

Q–17

Women's Health/Reproductive

Which of the following antibiotics is known to cause fetal harm if given to a pregnant woman?

(A) Azithromycin
(B) Clindamycin
(C) Gentamicin
(D) Ceftriaxone

Your Answer _____

Q–18

EENT

Emergent management of epiglottitis in children includes all of the following EXCEPT

(A) Place the child in an upright position and keep the child calm.
(B) Appropriate management of respiratory distress.
(C) Immediate examination of the pharynx to identify the swollen epiglottis and confirm the diagnosis.
(D) Alert a team of professionals for placement of an endotracheal tube.

Your Answer _____

Correct Answers

A–17

(C) Gentamicin and other aminoglycosides may be oto-toxic to a fetus. The other drugs listed have no overt toxicity reported to date.

A–18

(C) Epiglottitis is a life-threatening infection characterized by an inflamed and edematous epiglottis. Emergent management includes positioning the child in an upright position in a quiet place where there is immediate access to necessary interventions, if needed, and keeping the child calm. Examination of the pharynx should be done only if there is a low probability of epiglottitis. When the diagnosis is likely given the child's history, you should defer the pharynx examination. Management of a compromised airway and respiratory distress may be needed.

Questions

Cardiovascular

A 67-year-old female presents to the clinic for her physical exam. On cardiac auscultation you hear a grade 3/6 holostystolic murmur at the left lower sternal border with radiation to the left upper sternal border. The murmur increases with inspiration. This is a description of which murmur?

(A) Aortic valve stenosis
(B) Mitral valve stenosis
(C) Pulmonary valve regurgitation
(D) Tricuspid valve regurgitation

Your Answer _____

_____

General Medicine/Radiology

Increased whiteness on a CT scan is referred to as "hyperdensity" or high attenuation. All of the following are causes of hyperdensities EXCEPT

(A) calcification
(B) ossification
(C) acute hemorrhage
(D) fat

Your Answer _____

_____

Correct Answers

A–19

(D) The murmur of aortic stenosis is a crescendo/decrescendo systolic murmur best heard over the right sternal border with radiation to the carotid arteries. Mitral valve stenosis is a diastolic, decrescendo murmur best heard at the cardiac apex in the left lateral decubitus position. Mitral valve stenosis may be associated with an opening snap. The murmur associated with pulmonary valve regurgitation is a diastolic, decrescendo murmur best heard over the left lower sternal border. The murmur described in the clinical scenario describes tricuspid valve regurgitation.

A–20

(D) Fat shows as increased darkness and is referred to as "hypodensity" or low attenuation. All the others show as hyperdensities.

Questions

Neurology/Radiology

Subarachnoid hemorrhage is most often due to

(A) a ruptured aneurysm
(B) laceration of the middle meningeal artery
(C) trauma
(D) either (A) or (C)

Your Answer _____

Musculoskeletal

All of the following deformities are associated with rheumatoid arthritis EXCEPT

(A) Heberden's node
(B) swan-neck
(C) boutonnière deformity
(D) ulnar deviation

Your Answer _____

Correct Answers

A–21

(D) Subarachnoid hemorrhage most often follows trauma to the head or a ruptured aneurysm. An acute epidural hematoma may result from laceration of the middle meningeal artery (choice B).

A–22

(A) Heberden's nodes may be found with osteoarthritis. The other choices occur in patients with a diagnosis of rheumatoid arthritis.

Questions

Anatomy/Musculoskeletal

When examining the knee, an anterior and posterior *drawer test* is used to identify

(A) a torn medial meniscus

(B) a torn lateral meniscus

(C) instability of the lateral and medial collateral ligaments

(D) instability of the anterior and posterior cruciate ligaments

Your Answer _____

Orthopedics/Musculoskeletal

A positive *drawer sign* is present if the examiner demonstrates

(A) the presence of fluid in the knee when the patella is moved greater than 3 mm in either an anterior or posterior direction.

(B) any palpable or audible click, grinding, or limited extension of the knee.

(C) a locking of the knee with anterior or posterior movement of the tibia.

(D) anterior or posterior movement of the knee greater than 5 mm in either direction.

Your Answer _____

Correct Answers

A–23

(D) The *drawer test* is used to assess instability of the anterior and posterior cruciate ligaments. The *McMurray* test is used to detect a torn medial or lateral meniscus. Abduction and adduction stress, also known as Valgus and Varus stress tests, are used to identify instability of the lateral and medial collateral ligaments.

A–24

(D) Answers (A), (B), and (C) may be indicative of knee problems, but they are not used to assess instability of the cruciate ligaments.

Questions

Cardiovascular

Which factor could result in the recording of a FALSELY ELEVATED blood pressure?

(A) Sphygmomanometer bladder in excess of 100% of arm circumference
(B) Concurrent use of long-acting nitrate medication
(C) Both
(D) Neither

Your Answer _____

Musculoskeletal

A 2-year-old child presents to your clinic holding her left arm close to her body, slightly pronated. The child's parents had been swinging the child by her arms when the child started crying. What is the best intervention?

(A) Obtain X-rays of the elbow looking for a sail sign.
(B) Obtain X-rays of both arms for comparison views.
(C) Place pressure on the radial head and with the other hand, supinate the forearm and flex the elbow.
(D) Place pressure on the radial head and with the other hand, supinate the forearm and extend the elbow.

Your Answer _____

Correct Answers

A–25

(D) Neither of the choices is associated with a falsely elevated blood pressure reading. Using a blood pressure cuff that is too big for the patient's arm may give a falsely low reading while using a cuff that is too narrow for the patient's arm will result in a falsely elevated reading. A patient taking long-acting nitrates may have decreased venous return and a lowering of blood pressure.

A–26

(C) This scenario describes nursemaids elbow. It is most common between the ages of 1 and 4 and it is a subluxation of the radial head when the forearm is pulled while the forearm is pronated and the elbow is extended. Diagnosis and treatment is obtained by reducing the radial head. In the hyperpronation method of reduction, the examiner places his or her finger on the radial head, and, with the opposite hand, supinates the forearm and flexes the elbow in one motion. X-rays are not necessary unless the reduction maneuver is not effective.

Questions

General Medicine question
applicable to any system

The difference between a patient screening interview and an assessment interview is that

(A) the goal of a screening interview is to find out if a problem exists while the goal of the assessment interview is to discover more about a defined problem.

(B) the screening interview places emphasis on past medical history while the assessment interview emphasizes the chief complaint.

(C) the screening interview is associated with a specific set of questions, e.g., CAGE or CRAFFT, while the assessment interview encompasses the entire medical history.

(D) there is no difference between a screening and an assessment interview.

Your Answer _____

_____

Correct Answers

A–27

(A) There is a difference between a screening interview and an assessment interview in that a screening interview attempts to find out if a problem exists. This is particularly true of CAGE, CRAFFT, TACE, and other questionnaires. The screening interview is only the start, and assessment goes on from there, i.e., defining the problem and coming to a definitive diagnosis.

Questions

Neurology

Symptoms of Bell's palsy include all of the following EXCEPT

(A) Inability to close the eyelid
(B) Unilateral facial droop
(C) Loss of sensation on the affected side
(D) Smoothing of forehead wrinkles

Your Answer _____

_____

Cardiovascular

Pulse pressure is defined as

(A) the backflow of blood to the vena cava during right atrial contraction.
(B) the lowest point to which the diastolic blood pressure falls.
(C) the difference between systolic and diastolic pressures.
(D) the systolic force exerted against the wall of arteries.

Your Answer _____

_____

Correct Answers

A–28

(C) Bell's palsy is an acute peripheral nerve palsy that affects the facial nerve. Those with Bell's palsy typically complain of weakness or paralysis of the muscles on the affected side of the face. The nasolabial fold and forehead smoothes, and the corner of the mouth droops. The eyelid does not close and the lower lid sags, leading to irritation of the eye and corneal ulcerations. Bell's palsy is often idiopathic but is also associated with HSV-1 and Lyme disease. Central nervous system lesions can cause a facial nerve palsy but it is forehead sparing. The facial nerve does not have any sensory nerve fibers, thus sensation to the affected side is preserved.

A–29

(C) The blood pressure falls to its lowest point during diastole and the systolic pressure is the force exerted against the wall of the arteries when the ventricles contract. A backflow of blood to the vena cava during right atrial contraction is the most prominent component of the jugular venous *pulse,* the "a" wave. This pulse can be visualized but not palpated.

Questions

Women's Health

All of the following statements about uterine leiomyomas are true EXCEPT

(A) they represent localized proliferation of smooth muscle cells surrounded by compressed muscle fibers.
(B) they represent a common clinical finding in women.
(C) they represent a pre-malignant uterine cancer.
(D) they are hormonally responsive to estrogen.

Your Answer _____

_____

Women's Health

Which of the following is/are (a) potential factor(s) in development of cervical neoplasia?

(A) Cigarette smoking
(B) Multiple sex partners
(C) Oral contraceptive use
(D) All of the above

Your Answer _____

_____

Correct Answers

A–30

(C) Leiomyomas are benign tumors that are present in approximately 30% of American women. The incidence increases with age and as many as 50% of women have this condition after age 40.

A–31

(D) (A), (B), and (C) have been shown to increase the chance of developing cervical carcinoma. Recent research is showing that use of oral contraceptives in the absence of other risk factors may not contribute to the development of carcinoma; however, the research is not yet complete.

Questions

Q–32

Women's Health

The most common reproductive tract malignancy in women is

(A) cervical cancer
(B) ovarian cancer
(C) endometrial cancer
(D) vulvar cancer

Your Answer _____

Q–33

Women's Health

The most common malignancy in women in developed countries is

(A) breast
(B) cervical
(C) lung
(D) uterine

Your Answer _____

Correct Answers

A–32

(C) Endometrial carcinoma is the most common genital tract malignancy and the fourth most common cancer in women. In 2013, 49,560 new cases were diagnosed in the United States. New cases of ovarian cancer in 2013 were 22,240; cervical cancer, 12,340; and vulvar cancer 4,700.

A–33

(A) Breast cancer is the most common cancer in women in developed countries. Cervical cancer ranks as the second most common gynecological cancer, but lung cancer is rated second most common overall. Uterine cancer ranks fourth in occurrence for all women.

Questions

Women's Health

Women with molar pregnancy may present with findings consistent with pregnancy. Which one of the following symptoms is the most characteristic of a molar pregnancy?

(A) Uterine size/dates discrepancy
(B) Painless bleeding
(C) Passage of tissue
(D) Exaggerated "morning sickness"

Your Answer _____

_____

Women's Health

Because of controversy surrounding hormone replacement therapy, many women are seeking alternative therapy for symptoms of menopause. Which of the following have proven to be successful treatment for the majority of women?

(A) Soy products
(B) SNRI antidepressants
(C) Antiseizure medications, e.g., gabapentin
(D) None of the above

Your Answer _____

_____

Correct Answers

(B) All answer choices are characteristic symptoms of molar pregnancy, but painless bleeding is the most characteristic and occurs in most patients early in the second trimester of the pregnancy.

(D) All answer choices can be suggested for possible management of hot flushes, but none have been proven successful for all women or for other symptom management.

Questions

Women's Health

Which of the following is/are (a) typical symptom(s) of molimina?

(A) Fluid retention
(B) Fluctuations in mood
(C) Food cravings
(D) All of the above

Your Answer _____

_____

Women's Health/Reproductive

Infertility is generally defined as failure

(A) to conceive after one year of unprotected sexual intercourse in women under 35 years of age
(B) to conceive after 18 months of unprotected sexual intercourse
(C) to conceive within 6 months of oral contraceptive use
(D) to carry repeated pregnancies to 8 weeks' gestation

Your Answer _____

_____

Correct Answers

A–36

(D) Many women experience peri-menstrual symptoms. In addition to the answer choices, some report anxiety, nervousness, variations in sexual feelings, and difficulty sleeping.

A–37

(A) Failure to conceive following one year of unprotected sexual intercourse is defined as infertility.

Questions

Women's Health/Reproductive

A woman's last menstrual period is dated from the

(A) first day of the last bleeding episode
(B) first day of the last "normal" period
(C) last day of the last "normal" period
(D) last day of the last bleeding episode

Your Answer _____

_____

Women's Health/Reproductive

The abbreviation of an obstetric history is often depicted as G(a), P(b,c,d,e). In such a recording, the $\underline{c}$ stands for the number of

(A) pregnancies
(B) living children
(C) abortions
(D) preterm pregnancies

Your Answer _____

_____

Correct Answers

A–38

(B) The first day of the last "normal" period is the date from which a woman's last menstrual period is measured. This is important in assessing gestational age in order to estimate the date of delivery. This information helps in managing possible preterm labor or postdates pregnancy as well as timing of specific evaluations throughout the pregnancy.

A–39

(D) The number of preterm pregnancies (20 through 36 weeks) is designated by the letter "c." The letter "a" refers to the number of pregnancies; "b" to the number of term pregnancies (beyond 36 weeks); "d" to the number of abortions and ectopic pregnancies; and "e" to the number of living children.

Questions

EENT

Uncomplicated acute sinusitis is often successfully treated without the use of antibiotics. Of the drug types listed, which one is contraindicated in acute sinusitis?

(A) Decongestants
(B) Antihistamines
(C) Intranasal steroids
(D) Analgesics

Your Answer _____

_____

EENT

You see a patient who gives a history of self-diagnosed acute sinusitis for three weeks. The patient has a temperature of 104°F and appears toxic. He has lid edema, proptosis, chemosis, and 3rd, 4th, and 6th cranial nerve palsies. He also has papilledema. The most likely diagnosis at this time is

(A) ethmoidal sinusitis
(B) orbital cellulitis
(C) septic cavernous sinus thrombophlebitis
(D) subdural empyema

Your Answer _____

_____

Correct Answers

A–40

(B) Antihistamines can thicken secretions, dry mucous membranes, and impair drainage. Decongestants decrease swelling in the mucous membranes of the nasal passage and improve breathing. Intranasal steroids are not necessary in most patients but may accelerate symptomatic improvement in some. Analgesics are helpful in relieving sinusitis associated pain.

A–41

(C) Septic cavernous sinus thrombophlebitis is the most likely diagnosis, due to elevated temperature and clinical manifestations. Orbital cellulitis would not typically cause cranial nerve palsies. Ethmoidal sinusitis implies containment of the infection within the ethmoid sinus. A subdural empyema may result from direct spread of the infection through bone or through venous channels. Clinical findings vary but may include personality changes, headaches, and alterations of consciousness.

Questions

Infectious Disease/EENT

The primary diagnostic method to distinguish acute otitis media from serous otitis media with effusion is

(A) needle aspiration of the middle ear
(B) tympanoplasty
(C) pneumatic otoscopy
(D) visual otoscopic examination

Your Answer _____

_____

EENT

You see a patient who complains of ear pain and pruritis. Inspection of the affected ear reveals inflammation and crusting in the canal. The patient experiences pain when you manipulate the external ear. The most likely diagnosis is

(A) otitis media
(B) otitis externa
(C) mastoiditis
(D) cerumen impaction

Your Answer _____

_____

Correct Answers

A–42

(C) Pneumatic otoscopy is performed to evaluate how well the eardrum responds to changes in pressure. Poor eardrum response to pressure changes indicates fluid in the middle ear, which prevents the eardrum and middle ear bones from moving properly and causes a corresponding impairment of hearing. Needle aspiration is used to confirm a diagnosis of purulent otitis media and to identify the causative organism. Tympanoplasty is reconstructive surgery of the tympanic membrane. A simple visual otoscopic examination may not be sufficient to differentiate the conditions.

A–43

(B) The signs and symptoms described are typical for otitis externa. Otitis media is not painful with manipulation of the external ear. Mastoiditis is infection of the part of the temporal bone located behind the ear. It is painful if pressure is applied to the mastoid process. Cerumen impaction does not cause crusting but rather the ear canal is filled with wax.

Questions

EENT

Which of the following clinical criteria have been proposed as suggestive of group A streptococcal pharyngitis?

(A) Tonsillar exudates
(B) Tender anterior adenopathy
(C) History of fever
(D) All of the above

Your Answer _____

EENT

Also known as "quinsy throat," this disorder is a complication of streptococcal tonsillitis most often seen in adolescents and young adults. The disorder is

(A) retropharyngeal infection
(B) peritonsillar abscess
(C) epiglottitis
(D) Ludwig's angina

Your Answer _____

Correct Answers

A–44

(D) All the choices are suggestive of group A streptococcal pharyngitis, but there is considerable overlap between streptococcal and viral pharyngitis. A throat culture can be obtained to identify group A streptococcus.

A–45

(B) Peritonsillar abscess is primarily due to group A streptococcal infection and presents as dysphagia, drooling, and a "hot potato voice." Retropharyngeal infections are most common in childhood, and epiglottitis is most seen in children between the ages of two and eight years. Ludwig's angina is cellulitis of the submandibular, submental, and sublingual areas and is due to a dental infection.

Questions

Q–46

EENT

The incidence of acute epiglottitis in children is decreasing due to immunization with

(A) DTaP
(B) PCV
(C) Influenza
(D) Hib

Your Answer _____

Q–47

Pediatrics

At what age should immunization against Hepatitis B begin in a baby who is NOT high risk?

(A) Birth
(B) Three months
(C) Six months
(D) Eighteen months

Your Answer _____

Correct Answers

A–46

(D) Epiglottis is most commonly caused by *Haemophilus influenza* type b. Therefore, vaccination with Hib has led to a decreased incidence of this serious and sometimes deadly infection. DTaP is a vaccine for prevention of diphtheria, tetanus, and pertussis. PCV is the pneumococcal vaccine, and the influenza vaccine is administered to prevent influenza.

A–47

(A) Hepatitis B vaccination is routinely given to all infants at birth.

Questions

Psychiatry

An 83-year-old female presents to the clinic with her family, concerned about weight loss, increased fatigue, and decreased interest in her favorite activities. You and her family are concerned about depression. Which of the following is false regarding geriatric depression?

(A) Depression is a normal part of aging.
(B) SSRI medications are associated with an increased risk of GI bleeding.
(C) Early dementia may present as depression.
(D) Depression increases following a myocardial infarction.

Your Answer _____

_____

Dermatology/Oncology

The most common cancer in the United States is

(A) skin
(B) lung
(C) breast
(D) colon

Your Answer _____

_____

Correct Answers

A–48

(A) Depression in the geriatric population is not a normal part of aging and may represent a relapse of depression from earlier in life, a cerebrovascular event, or the onset of dementia. Depression is also more frequent following a stroke or myocardial infarction. Symptoms of depression in the older adult include weight loss, fatigue, and hypersomnolence. These symptoms may be falsely attributed to medical comorbidities or medication side effects. Side effects of SSRIs include serotonin syndrome, hyponatremia, falls, fractures, and GI bleeding. SSRIs must be used carefully in case of decreased renal or hepatic function and/or polypharmacy.

A–49

(A) Nonmelanoma skin cancer is the most common cancer in the U.S., with more than 3.5 million new cases diagnosed annually. The second, third, and fourth most frequent cancers in the U.S. are lung, prostate, and breast.

Questions

Oncology

The most common cancer in women worldwide is

(A) breast
(B) bowel
(C) lung
(D) stomach

Your Answer _____

Internal Medicine/General Medicine

Fever is characterized by

(A) a failure in thermal control mechanisms
(B) a rise in the hypothalamic thermal set point
(C) an excess in heat dissipation
(D) All of the above

Your Answer _____

Correct Answers

A–50

(A) The most common cancer for women worldwide is breast cancer. The most common cancers for men worldwide are lung and bronchus.

A–51

(B) In fever, the hypothalamic thermal set point rises and is a condition best treated by drugs such as aspirin, acetaminophen, or other COX inhibitors. Hyperthermia is caused by a failure of thermoregulation such that heat production exceeds heat dissipation.

Questions

Internal Medicine

Hyperthermia is characterized by

(A) a failure in thermal control mechanisms
(B) a rise in the hypothalamic thermal set point
(C) an excess in heat dissipation
(D) all of the above

Your Answer _____

_____

Emergency Medicine

The most common hyperthermic emergency is due to

(A) malignant hyperthermia of anesthesia
(B) classic heatstroke
(C) neuroleptic syndrome
(D) excessive sweating

Your Answer _____

_____

Correct Answers

A–52

(A) Hyperthermia is caused by a failure of thermoregulation such that heat production exceeds heat dissipation. *Fever* is associated with a rise in the hypothalamic thermal set point.

A–53

(B) Classic heatstroke is the most common hyperthermic emergency, and it occurs principally during summer heat waves. It is most likely to affect the elderly and patients with serious underlying diseases. Both (A) and (C) are also causes of hyperthermia but occur less frequently than heatstroke. Sweating is one way of dissipating heat.

Questions

Neurology

A patient with Parkinson's Disease stopped taking his levodopa and amantadine. His wife brought him to the clinic and reported that over the past three days her husband had exhibited bradykinesia, severe muscular rigidity, altered sensorium, and diaphoresis. His heart rate averaged 110 beats per minute and his blood pressure had been labile. Laboratory tests showed hemoconcentration, leukocytosis, rhabdomyolysis, and mild acidosis. Which of the following would be very high on your differential diagnosis?

(A) Serotonin syndrome
(B) Neuroleptic malignant syndrome
(C) Hyperthermia
(D) Lethal catatonia

Your Answer _____

_____

Correct Answers

(B) Neuroleptic malignant syndrome (NMS) would be suspected due to the abrupt withdrawal of anti-Parkinson drugs. NMS is thought to be due to a blockade of dopaminergic receptors in the nigrostriatal tracts or from sudden lack of dopamine availability. In this case, the severe muscular rigidity probably led to excessive heat production with the subsequent abnormal laboratory findings. Serotonin syndrome begins abruptly and is most often encountered in patients taking SSRIs or other antidepressants or by drug interactions while on these medications. Lethal catatonia is an uncommon psychiatric disorder in which agitation progresses to muscular rigidity and hyperthermia. It may be confused with NMS; however, NMS has been found to be directly related to an abrupt discontinuation of anti-Parkinson medications.

Questions

Surgery

The most frequently used method of controlling fertility used in the United States is

(A) sterilization
(B) oral contraceptives
(C) tubal ligation
(D) vaginal hysterectomy

Your Answer _____

Surgery

Success rates for a healthy pregnancy following reversal of fallopian tube ligation are reported to be between

(A) 75–100%
(B) 20–70%
(C) 10–50%
(D) 5–7%

Your Answer _____

Correct Answers

A–55

(B) Oral contraceptives are the most frequently used method of controlling fertility in the United States, but most women are able to conceive following their discontinuation. Sterilization provides an absolute method of controlling fertility. Tubal ligation is a reversible method of contraception. Vaginal hysterectomy was once a preferred means of permanent sterilization but is rarely used today.

A–56

(B) Success rates for a healthy pregnancy following reversal of tubal ligation approach 20–70%. However, there is an increased risk of ectopic pregnancy in women undergoing such procedures.

Questions

Women's Health

The normal vaginal pH range of women during their reproductive age is

(A) 6.5–8.5
(B) 3.5–4.5
(C) 5.0–7.0
(D) 2.0–3.0

Your Answer _____

_____

Reproductive

You see a 28-year-old woman with a complaint of vaginitis. On physical examination, you observe a copious "frothy" discharge with a rancid odor along with petechiae in the upper vagina and on the cervix. Your most likely diagnosis is

(A) candidiasis
(B) bacterial vaginosis
(C) gonorrhea
(D) trichomoniasis

Your Answer _____

_____

Correct Answers

A–57

(B) Women during their reproductive years have a vaginal pH between 3.5 and 4.5. Before puberty and after menopause, the vaginal pH ranges from 6–8.

A–58

(D) The description fits most closely with a diagnosis of trichomoniasis. Candidiasis presents with a white, "cottage cheese-like" discharge; bacterial vaginosis with a thin, gray to white, adherent discharge and a fishy odor. Gonorrhea causes a malodorous, purulent discharge which may be overlooked by the patient until pelvic infection occurs.

Questions

Infectious Disease

The most common sexually transmitted bacterial disease is

(A) *Chlamydia trachomatis*
(B) *Neisseria gonorrhoeae*
(C) *Herpes simples,* Type 2
(D) HIV/AIDS

Your Answer _____

Infectious Disease

You have an 18-year-old hospitalized patient with confirmed pelvic inflammatory disease secondary to *Neisseria gonorrhea.* Your initial therapy should be

(A) streptomycin 500 mg every 12 hours
(B) doxycycline 100 mg every 12 hours
(C) ceftriaxone 250 mg IM every 12 hours plus doxycycline 100 mg P.O. every 12 hours
(D) cefoxitin 2 g IV every 6 hours plus doxycycline 100 mg IV every 12 hours

Your Answer _____

Correct Answers

A–59

(A) *Chlamydia trachomatis* is the most common sexually transmitted bacterial disease. The most common STI overall is HPV.

A–60

(D) Patients sick enough to require hospitalization would more likely be treated with cefoxitin plus doxycycline. Choice (C) is more commonly used in an outpatient. Neither (A) nor (B), as single therapy, is recommended in pelvic inflammatory disease.

Questions

Infectious Disease

Which of the following statements about the human papillomavirus is/are correct?

(A) It is a DNA virus.
(B) It is species specific and only infects humans.
(C) Sequelae of HPV infection may take years to develop.
(D) All of the above are correct.

Your Answer _____

Infectious Disease

The chancre of primary syphilis develops approximately 10–90 days after infection with *Treponema pallidum.* If left untreated, the ulcer will heal and secondary syphilis may develop within

(A) 4–8 weeks after the primary chancre first appears
(B) 2–3 weeks after the primary chancre first appears
(C) 1–10 years after the primary infection
(D) 6 months after the primary infection

Your Answer _____

Correct Answers

A–61

(D) All the statements are true.

A–62

(A) Four to eight weeks after the primary chancre appears, manifestations of secondary syphilis occur.

Questions

Dermatology

Fournier's gangrene is a necrotizing fasciitis of the groin and perineum. All of the following are true regarding management of Fournier's gangrene EXCEPT

(A) Antibiotic therapy without surgical debridement is associated with almost a 100% mortality rate.
(B) Repeated surgeries are often necessary.
(C) Antibiotic coverage should cover gram-positive, gram-negative, and anaerobic organisms.
(D) Hyperbaric oxygen therapy is indicated as initial therapy in place of antibiotic and surgical debridement.

Your Answer _____

_____

Anatomy

Uterine procidentia describes a condition whereby the

(A) uterus descends beyond the vulva
(B) urethra becomes detached from the endopelvic fascia
(C) small bowel herniates through the vaginal wall
(D) uterus prolapses

Your Answer _____

_____

Correct Answers

A–63

(D) Treatment of Fournier's gangrene includes antibiotics that cover gram-positive, gram-negative, and anaerobes in addition to surgical debridement. In fact, surgical debridement is a mainstay of treatment. Hyperbaric oxygen therapy can also be a part of treatment but is not used in place of surgical debridement or IV antibiotic therapy.

A–64

(A) When the uterus descends beyond the vulva, it is termed uterine procidentia.

Questions

Urology

All of the following are surgical procedures used in treating urinary incontinence EXCEPT the

(A) Burch suspension
(B) S-lift
(C) Kelly-Kennedy procedure
(D) Marshall-Marchetti-Krantz procedure

Your Answer _____

Infectious Disease

In laboratory evaluation of a patient suspected of having a urinary tract infection, cultures of urine samples that show colony counts of more than _____ for a single organism generally indicate infection.

(A) 10,000
(B) 50,000
(C) 100,000
(D) 500,000

Your Answer _____

Correct Answers

A–65

(B) The S-lift is a mini-facelift that provides an overall lift to the neck and lower third of the face.

A–66

(C) Colony counts of more than 100,000 for a single organism generally indicate infection. However, counts as low as 10,000 for *E. coli* are associated with infection when symptoms are present.

Questions

Women's Health

Endometriosis is a common finding in women with infertility and it has various clinical presentations. The "gold standard" in making a diagnosis of endometriosis is

(A) a complete medical history
(B) a complete physical examination
(C) a CT scan of the pelvic floor
(D) none of the above

Your Answer _____

_____

Surgery

Extirpative surgery for endometriosis is reserved for which kind of cases?

(A) Women who wish to become pregnant in the future.
(B) Women whose disease is very extensive.
(C) Women who have completed their family and wish definitive therapy.
(D) Both (B) and (C) are cases for extirpative surgery.

Your Answer _____

_____

Correct Answers

A–67

(D) Precisely because of the diverse presentations of endometriosis, establishing a diagnosis requires direct visualization of the lesions either at the time of laparoscopy or via tissue biopsy.

A–68

(D) Extirpative or definitive surgery is reserved only for cases in which the disease is so extensive that conservative therapy is not feasible and there is a presence of intractable pelvic pain or in women who have completed their family and wish definitive therapy.

Questions

Women's Health

A 27-year-old woman presents with a spontaneous bloody nipple discharge. She has no previous personal history or family history of breast cancer. The most likely diagnosis is

(A) mastalgia
(B) fibroadenoma
(C) cancer
(D) intraductal papilloma

Your Answer _____

_____

Surgery

An endometrial ablation refers to

(A) a surgical procedure to destroy the endometrial lining to reduce menstrual bleeding
(B) a procedure to evaluate the surface of the cervix when malignancy is suspected
(C) the delivery of highly energetic light beams to the endometrium to facilitate tissue destruction
(D) the passage of a small, hollow tube through the cervix with subsequent aspiration of endometrial tissue for examination

Your Answer _____

_____

Correct Answers

A–69

(D) Intraductal papillomas are fibrovascular tumors arising in the ducts of the breast. The patient presents with a spontaneous bloody, serous, or cloudy nipple discharge. Mastalgia refers to pain in the breast. A fibroadenoma is usually a solitary lesion that is slow growing that may need excision but often is managed medically. Breast cancers most often present as a mass initially, and discharge is a late occurrence associated with poor prognosis.

A–70

(A) Answer (B) refers to a colposcopy, (C) to laser vaporization, and (D) to endometrial biopsy.

Questions

Psychiatry

To treat a psychiatric patient effectively, the interviewer must make a reliable and accurate diagnosis. Which of the following interviewing skills/techniques would be appropriate in interacting with such a patient?

(A) Question the patient in terms of genetic, temperamental, biological, developmental, social, and psychological influences in his/her life.

(B) Placing chairs without any furniture between the clinician and the patient.

(C) Leaving the door to an interview room open.

(D) All of the above are appropriate techniques when interviewing a psychiatric patient.

Your Answer _____

_____

Correct Answers

(D) Depending upon the presentation of the patient, all of the mentioned techniques may be useful. The clinician must learn as much as possible about the patient while building trust with the patient. The manner in which furniture is arranged helps to build trust. For example, the chairs should be of equal height so neither person looks down on the other. If the patient is potentially dangerous, it is appropriate to leave the door to the interview room open and even to post a third individual outside or even inside the door. For legal and medical reasons, an adequate written record of the patient's treatment must be maintained. Taking notes during the interview is also appropriate.

Questions

Women's Health

A *peau d'orange* appearance of the skin of the breast indicates

(A) edema of breast caused by blocked lymph drainage
(B) advanced or inflammatory carcinoma
(C) previous radiation treatments for breast cancer
(D) both (A) and (B) are correct answers

Your Answer _____

Psychiatry

Which of the following procedures can be used to induce a panic attack in a patient with panic disorder?

(A) Dexamethasone Suppression Test
(B) Ice-water lavage
(C) Lactate provocation
(D) Have the patient eat a banana, avocado, or other foods high in serotonin.

Your Answer _____

Correct Answers

A–72

(D) A *peau d'orange* discoloration of the breast indicates carcinoma and is caused by blockage of lymph drainage. Previous radiation of the skin as needed for treatment of breast cancer may result in redness of the skin.

A–73

(C) Up to 72% of patients with panic disorder have a panic attack when administered an IV injection of sodium lactate. This test may also be used to trigger flashbacks in patients with post-traumatic stress disorder.

Questions

Psychiatry

Which of the following substances can be detected by a urine drug screen?

(A) Amphetamines
(B) Marijuana
(C) Barbiturates
(D) All of the above

Your Answer _____

Psychiatry

Which of the following statements most closely identifies *delirium?*

(A) An unpleasant mood
(B) Inability or difficulty in describing or being aware of one's emotions or mood
(C) Bewildered, confused, disoriented reaction associated with fear and hallucination
(D) Increased motor and psychological activity that is unpleasant

Your Answer _____

Correct Answers

A–74

(D) All the substances can be detected by a urine drug screen. Accuracy of the test, however, depends on the length of time since the patient encountered the substance.

A–75

(C) Response (A) describes dysphoria; response (B) describes alexithymia, and response (D) is descriptive of tension.

Questions

Neurology

Which of the following best describes absence seizures?

(A) No disruption in consciousness; onset during childhood; a partial seizure

(B) Consciousness is interrupted; manifested by isolated jerks; onset during childhood

(C) Onset in childhood; disruption of consciousness; no convulsive movements

(D) A generalized seizure; onset in early adulthood; convulsive movements present

Your Answer _____

Neurology

Multiple sclerosis is characterized by which of the following?

(A) Lesions are present in the white matter of the central nervous system.

(B) It is more common in men than women.

(C) It has an onset in the 40–50 age group.

(D) It is associated with cognitive symptoms but not with behavioral symptoms.

Your Answer _____

Correct Answers

A–76

(C) Absence (petit mal) seizures are a type of generalized seizure that usually begins between the ages of five and seven years and ceases by puberty. The patient has brief disruptions of consciousness but does not lose consciousness altogether. He/she may or may not have twitching of the eyes or slight jerking movements.

A–77

(A) Multiple sclerosis is characterized by many symptoms, pathophysiologically related to multifocal lesions in the white matter of the CNS. It is more common in women, with onset more often between the ages of 20 and 40 years. It is associated with both cognitive and behavioral symptoms.

Questions

Neurology

Creutzfeldt-Jakob disease is

(A) a degenerative brain disease thought to be caused by a prion infection

(B) a genetic disorder characterized by an accumulation of fatty acid derivatives in the brain

(C) an inherited neurological disease characterized by motor and sensory neuropathy

(D) a hereditary muscle disease that weakens the muscles that move the body

Your Answer _____

_____

Correct Answers

A-78

(A) Creutzfeldt-Jakob disease is a rare degenerative brain disease thought to be caused by a prion infection, although a definitive organism has not been identified in people with the disease. It usually first appears between ages 20 and 70, with the average age of the onset of symptoms in the late 50s, and death usually occurs within one year of diagnosis. Answer (B) is descriptive of Tay-Sachs disease and answer (C) of Charcot-Marie-Tooth disease. Answer (D) is descriptive of muscular dystrophy.

Questions

Gastroenterology/Neurology

A father brings in his 31-year-old son, Robert, who is apathetic. The father states that Robert sleeps all day and is awake at night. He further states that Robert has been drinking alcohol heavily for the past couple of years. On physical examination, you note asterixis, and the laboratory evaluation of ammonia is elevated. A diagnosis you must consider is

(A) Reye's syndrome
(B) uremic encephalopathy
(C) hepatic encephalopathy
(D) muscular exertion

Your Answer _____

Infectious Disease

Which of the following criteria may be used for a case definition of AIDS?

(A) CD4+ T cell counts <200/mm^3
(B) CD4+ T cell counts <14% of total T cells, regardless of symptomatology
(C) Presence of AIDS-related opportunistic infection
(D) Any of the above.

Your Answer _____

Correct Answers

A–79

(C) In this scenario, the most likely diagnosis is hepatic encephalopathy. Reye's syndrome is seen in children but may also cause an elevation in ammonia levels. There is no history to indicate uremic encephalopathy such as renal failure. Muscular exertion can elevate ammonium levels but would not be associated with asterixis.

A–80

(D) Either (A), (B), or (C) can be used for a case definition of AIDS.

Questions

Dermatologic

Kaposi's sarcoma is the most common type of malignancy present among homosexual or bisexual HIV-infected men. Evidence suggests that it is caused by a sexually transmitted agent other than HIV. That agent is thought to be

(A) herpes simplex virus type 2
(B) human herpes virus type 8
(C) Cytomegalovirus
(D) Epstein-Barr virus

Your Answer _____

Hematology

Anisocytosis refers to

(A) an abnormal variation in the size of red blood cells
(B) an abnormal variation in the shape of red blood cells
(C) Both
(D) Neither

Your Answer _____

Correct Answers

A–81

(B) Human herpes virus type 8 is thought to be the causative agent for Kaposi's sarcoma. Herpes simplex virus
type 2 causes genital or perianal ulcerations. It can be
spread by direct skin contact. Cytomegalovirus causes
disseminated disease and Epstein-Barr virus causes infectious mononucleosis.

A–82

(A) Anisocytosis refers to an abnormal variation in the
size of red blood cells. Poikilocytosis is the term that refers
to an abnormal shape of red blood cells.

Questions

Neurology

A good question to ask patients to assess their recent memory function is

(A) what is their date of birth
(B) what they ate for their last meal
(C) how many siblings they have
(D) what is 100 minus 6

Your Answer _____

_____

General Medicine

Which of the following mechanisms may cause edema?

(A) Increased hydrostatic pressure
(B) Increased permeability of blood vessels
(C) Decreased colloid osmotic pressure
(D) (A), (B), and (C) may cause edema

Your Answer _____

_____

Correct Answers

A–83

(B) Asking a patient what he/she ate for their last meal is a common way to evaluate recent memory. The other choices reflect old, well-learned information.

A–84

(D) All of the mentioned mechanisms may result in fluid accumulation in the tissues. Congestive heart failure may increase hydrostatic pressure; acute inflammation can increase permeability of blood vessels; and hypoalbumin-emia will decrease colloid osmotic pressure.

Questions

Genetics/General Medicine

All of the following are examples of autosomal dominant disorders EXCEPT

(A) albinism
(B) familial hypercholesterolemia
(C) von Willebrand's disease
(D) Marfan syndrome

Your Answer _____

_____

Gastrointestinal

Korsakoff's syndrome is caused by a lack of

(A) niacin
(B) riboflavin
(C) thiamine
(D) pyridoxine

Your Answer _____

_____

Correct Answers

A–85

(A) Albinism is an autosomal recessive disorder; all the rest represent an autosomal dominant inheritance pattern.

A–86

(C) A deficiency of thiamine will cause Korsakoff's syndrome. This syndrome is manifested by damage to neurons and supporting cells in the central nervous system.

Questions

Psychiatry

The most common type of hallucination experienced by a patient with schizophrenia is

(A) auditory
(B) visual
(C) tactile
(D) olfactory

Your Answer _____

_____

Pediatric/Orthopedics

The most common cause of hip pain in an adolescent is

(A) scoliosis
(B) slipped capital femoral epiphysis
(C) genu valgum
(D) tendon strains

Your Answer _____

_____

Correct Answers

A–87

(A) A patient with schizophrenia most often experiences auditory hallucinations or "hears voices" inside his/her head.

A–88

(B) A slipped capital femoral epiphysis or an apophyseal avulsion is the most common cause of hip pain in an adolescent. Severe genu valgum, aka "knock-knees," may cause hip discomfort with severe cases, but the severe form is relatively infrequent in its occurrence. In adults, hip pain more often occurs secondary to tendon strains and arthritis. Scoliois is a skeletal deformity of the spine.

Questions

General Medicine/Genetics

Which of the following statements is NOT characteristic of X-linked recessive inheritance?

(A) The mutant gene is on an X chromosome.
(B) Males are more commonly affected than females.
(C) No father-to-son transmission exists.
(D) Half of the daughters of an affected father and a normal mother will be carriers.

Your Answer _____

General Medicine/Genetics

Which one of the following karyotypes represents Klinefelter's syndrome?

(A) 47, XX, +21 or 47, XY, +21
(B) 45, X or 45, XO
(C) 47, XXY or 46, XY/47, XXY
(D) t(9;22)

Your Answer _____

Correct Answers

A–89

(D) All the daughters of an affected father and a normal mother will be carriers because the father will pass on the X chromosome to each.

A–90

(C) Klinefelter's syndrome is a condition that occurs in males who have an extra X chromosome in most of their cells and is represented by the karyotype depicted in choice (C). Choice (A) depicts Down syndrome; choice (B) depicts Turner syndrome; and choice (D) represents a structural disorder caused by translocation between chromosomes 9 and 22.

Questions

Pediatrics

The C in TORCH stands for

(A) cystic fibrosis
(B) cytomegalovirus
(C) chlamydia
(D) *Clostridium difficile*

Your Answer _____

EENT

All of the following are true regarding hearing loss screening EXCEPT

(A) Asymptomatic adults >50 years old should be screened every 3 years.
(B) Whispered voice, finger rub, and watch tick tests are preferred screening tests in adults.
(C) All infants should have a hearing screening test before 1 month of age.
(D) Otoacoustic emissions is the preferred screening test in infants.

Your Answer _____

Correct Answers

A–91

(B) The C stands for cytomegalovirus, one of the infectious teratogens. The others are: T = Toxoplasmosis; O = Other (hepatitis B, HIV); R = Rubella; H = Herpes Simplex.

A–92

(A) Newborn hearing screening is performed using otoacoustic emissions (OAEs) followed by a confirmatory test, auditory brainstem response (ABR). All infants should be screened by 1 month of age and a diagnosis of hearing loss should be made by 3 months of age. There are no recommended screening guidelines for adults. Whispered voice, finger rub, and watch tick tests are all preferred screening tests and diagnosis can be made by an audiology evaluation.

Questions

Pediatrics

Which of the following are at high risk for developmental dysplasia of the hip?

(A) First born males, breech presentation
(B) First born females, breech presentation
(C) Premature birth, either sex
(D) Post-term infants

Your Answer _____

Pediatric/Orthopedics

Of the three primary causes of rotational "turning-in" or "pigeon-toed" deformities in children, which will spontaneously resolve in most cases?

(A) Curved feet (metatarsus adductus)
(B) Twisted shins (internal tibial torsion)
(C) Twisted thigh bones (femoral anteversion)
(D) All of the above

Your Answer _____

Correct Answers

A–93

(B) Females with a breech presentation are more susceptible to hip dysplasia.

A–94

(D) All of the mentioned rotational deformities usually resolve and reassurance of the parents is most helpful.

Questions

General Medicine

Which of the following has/have been identified as barriers to effective chronic disease care?

(A) Lack of patient trust in the medical provider
(B) Lack of understanding of treatment regimens
(C) Lack of provider time
(D) All of the above

Your Answer _____

Infectious Disease/Women's Health

A 26-year-old woman comes to your clinic for a Papanicolaou test and contraceptive discussion. She complains of mild dyspareunia. While doing the Pap smear you also collect a vaginal sample for culture to rule out gonorrhea and chlamydial infection. The culture was negative for both these organisms but *Escherichia coli* was reported. The patient denied symptoms of urinary tract infection or vaginitis. Should she be treated and, if so, with what drug?

(A) Yes, begin amoxicillin.
(B) Yes, begin trimethoprim/sulfisoxazole.
(C) Yes, begin OTC vaginal douche.
(D) No, treatment is unnecessary.

Your Answer _____

Correct Answers

A–95

(D) All of the answer choices are barriers to effective chronic disease care. Patients often do not trust their provider because of a perception that the provider is rushed and doesn't take time to listen effectively to the complaints of the patient. Thorough and accurate education should be provided to patients in order to promote compliance.

A–96

(D) There is no reason to treat asymptomatic vaginal colonization with *E. coli*. Colonization is very common in healthy women and there is no data indicating that treatment is beneficial. Vaginal douching is considered an unhealthy behavior that may lead to further infection and should not be encouraged by health care providers.

Questions

Women's Health

Which of the following descriptions of breast masses is consistent with fibrocystic disease?

(A) Firm, rubbery consistency
(B) Poorly delineated borders
(C) Tender to palpation
(D) No variation with menses

Your Answer _____

_____

General Medicine

Which of the following groups of drugs does NOT have independent analgesic activity?

(A) SSRIs
(B) Tricyclics
(C) SNRIs
(D) Anticonvulsants

Your Answer _____

_____

Correct Answers

A–97

(C) Fibrocystic breast disease is usually tender to palpation, and pain and tenderness increase premenstrually. Masses that are firm and rubbery are consistent with a diagnosis of fibroadenoma and those with poorly delineated, irregular borders are consistent with cancer.

A–98

(A) Selective Serotonin Reuptake Inhibitors (SSRIs) do not have independent analgesic activity as all of the others do.

Questions

Q–99

Psychiatry

Munchausen syndrome is classified as a(n)

(A) anxiety disorder
(B) adjustment disorder
(C) somatization disorder
(D) factitious disorder

Your Answer _____

Q–100

Musculoskeletal

You see a patient with radiographic evidence of osteoarthritis of the knee. Supporting clinical findings of knee joint pain, morning stiffness, decreased range of motion, and local swelling support your diagnosis. Which of the following labs would be most helpful in confirming your diagnosis?

(A) CBC
(B) Erythrocyte sedimentation rate
(C) C-reactive protein
(D) None are useful.

Your Answer _____

Correct Answers

A–99

(D) A factitious disorder is a mental disturbance in which a patient intentionally acts mentally or physically ill without any obvious signs or symptoms. Symptoms are either falsified or self-induced by the patient.

A–100

(D) All of the listed labs would be within normal limits if the diagnosis of osteoarthritis is correct. CBC is used to evaluate for infection, anemias, or other blood cell disorders. Erythrocyte sedimentation rate (ESR) is sometimes used to evaluate for rheumatoid arthritis. C-reactive protein is measured to indicate inflammation, such as in Rheumatoid Arthritis, autoimmune disease, and heart disease.

Questions

General Medicine/Dermatology

A 35-year-old woman presents with distal onycholysis of the fingers but denies any other symptoms. She denies recent outdoor activities such as gardening. What is your initial approach to identifying the cause of onycholysis?

(A) Order a bacterial culture
(B) Order a radiograph of the fingers
(C) Measure the patient's thyroxine level
(D) Measure the patient's TSH level

Your Answer _____

Dermatology

In performing a physical examination on a 28-year-old fair-skinned female, you note a single dark streak on the left forefinger nail. The patient denies trauma, pain, or other symptoms. Her family history is negative except for mild hypertension in her father. How would you proceed?

(A) Dismiss it as a variation of normal
(B) Perform a fungal culture
(C) Search the body for pigmented lesions
(D) Order a biopsy of the nail and underlying tissue

Your Answer _____

Correct Answers

A–101

(D) Onycholysis is the separation of the distal margin of the nail plate from the nail bed. This condition is seen in patients with hyperthyroidism and is referred to as Plummer's nails. Measurement of the TSH would provide an indication to the underlying pathology. This condition is also seen in patients with yeast or other infections as well as local trauma, but since there is no history of trauma, the most likely diagnosis is hyperthyroidism.

A–102

(D) A single streaked nail in a fair-skinned person may indicate melanoma or dysplastic nevus. In addition to performing a thorough dermatologic examination, the nail and underlying tissue should be biopsied.

Questions

Musculoskeletal

A 32-year-old man presents with a 10-day history of pain, swelling, and redness of the left elbow. He denies recent illness but notes that the problem with his elbow began after a fall while playing basketball. The impact of the fall was on his left elbow. Physical examination reveals a decrease in range of motion in all directions but more limitation with full flexion due to pain. The olecranon is tender to palpation. Radiographs of the elbow are normal. Your working diagnosis is

(A) lateral epicondylitis
(B) medial epicondylitis
(C) olecranon bursitis
(D) gouty arthritis

Your Answer _____

_____

Correct Answers

A–103

(C) Patients with bursitis typically have swelling, erythema, and localized pain over the affected bursa both at rest and with motion. Decreased range of motion may also be present. The history of acute trauma is important in differentiating bursitis from tendonitis. Epicondylitis is a painful inflammation of the muscles and soft tissues around the medial (golfer's elbow) or lateral (tennis elbow) epicondyle. It is brought on by overuse of the muscles. Gout is an arthritic condition caused by elevated levels of uric acid in the bloodstream. Crystals of uric acid precipitate in the joints and cause painful inflammation.

Questions

Musculoskeletal

"Tennis elbow" is the common name applied to

(A)   lateral epicondylitis
(B)   medial epicondylitis
(C)   olecranon bursitis
(D)   triceps tendinitis

Your Answer _____

_____

Musculoskeletal

When treating a patient with osteoporosis with oral bisphosphonates, a potential complication that must be monitored is

(A)   the development of myeloma
(B)   mandibular osteonecrosis
(C)   Paget's disease
(D)   renal tubular acidosis

Your Answer _____

_____

Correct Answers

A–104

(A) Lateral epicondylitis is a condition where the outer-part of the elbow becomes painful and tender. It is seen in persons playing tennis but may occur in anyone after repeated motion use of the elbow.

A–105

(B) Osteonecrosis of the mandible has emerged as a potential complication of bisphosphonate therapy. It is prudent to have your patient cleared by his/her dentist prior to beginning bisphosphonate therapy. There is an approxi-mately three times greater risk of osteonecrosis of the jaw in patients taking bisphosphonates than patients not taking the drugs. This may develop after dental extractions and implants, but it may also occur spontaneously.

Questions

Endocrinology

The American Diabetes Association has set goals for optimal management of diabetes and potential comorbidities. Which of the following represents those goals?

(A) Hemoglobin $A_{1c} \leq 6\%$; LDL Cholesterol ≤ 130 mg/dL; blood pressure $\leq 140/90$ mmHg

(B) Hemoglobin $A_{1c} \leq 7\%$; LDL Cholesterol ≤ 100 mg/dL; blood pressure $< 140/90$ mmHg

(C) Hemoglobin $A_{1c} \leq 6\%$; LDL Cholesterol ≤ 130 mg/dL; blood pressure $\leq 120/80$ mmHg

(D) Hemoglobin $A_{1c} \leq 8\%$; LDL Cholesterol ≤ 150 mg/dL; blood pressure $\leq 140/90$ mmHg

Your Answer _____

_____

Musculoskeletal

A positive Finkelstein's test is diagnostic for

(A) de Quervain tenosynovitis
(B) trochanteric bursitis
(C) iliotibial band syndrome
(D) meniscal injury

Your Answer _____

_____

Correct Answers

A–106

(B) Current recommendations are as stated for persons over age 40 who do not have active cardiovascular disease.

A–107

(A) De Quervain tenosynovitis is the inflammation of the tendons on the side of the wrist at the base of the thumb. Pain can be recreated when the thumb is folded across the palm and the fingers are flexed over the thumb followed by ulnar deviation of the wrist. This is a positive Finkelstein maneuver.

Questions

Q–108

Dermatology

Which of the following statements is true regarding ichthyosis?

(A)   Mildly pruritic; present during winter months only
(B)   Well-defined patches and plaques of scale and erythema
(C)   Asymptomatic, occurs year round, aggravated by dry weather
(D)   Petechial or pruritic eruption; may or may not be localized to the skin

Your Answer _____

Q–109

Dermatology

Koilonychia best describes nails with which appearance?

(A)   Infection of the nail fold
(B)   Atrophy of the nail plate
(C)   Brittle nails that often split vertically
(D)   Thin, concave nails with raised ridges

Your Answer _____

Correct Answers

A–108

(C) Ichthyosis is the term to describe severe, persistent problems with dry skin. This condition can range from very mild to life threatening.

A–109

(D) Koilonychia describes nails that are thin and concave (spoon nails) with horizontal ridges. They often result from iron deficiency anemia.

Questions

Hematology/Pharmacology

You have a patient who takes prednisone chronically. What effect will the prednisone have on the CBC?

(A) Leukocytosis
(B) Leukopenia
(C) Eosinophilia
(D) Lymphocytosis

Your Answer _____

Hematology

Which of the following conditions may cause an eosinophilia?

(A) Allergic reactions
(B) Parasitic infections
(C) Cushing's syndrome
(D) Both (A) and (B) are correct.

Your Answer _____

Correct Answers

A–110

(A) Corticosteroids, e.g., prednisone, increase blood levels of leukocytes causing leukocytosis. They decrease eosinophils, basophils, monocytes, and lymphocytes by redistributing them to lymphoid tissue from the circulation.

A–111

(D) The most common cause of eosinophilia worldwide is parasitic infections. Other conditions, such as allergies and certain tumors, may also increase eosinophils.

Questions

Hematology

Which one of the following conditions is most likely to cause a lymphocytosis?

(A) Lupus erythematosus
(B) HIV
(C) Mononucleosis
(D) Hodgkin's disease

Your Answer _____

Gastrointestinal

In a patient with achalasia, a barium swallow will show

(A) Schatzki rings
(B) protrusion of the stomach through the opening at the esophagus and/or the diaphragm
(C) dilation of the esophagus with a beaklike narrowing at the esophagogastric junction
(D) irregular borders and sharp angles of the esophagus

Your Answer _____

Correct Answers

A–112

(C) Viral infections, such as mononucleosis, are the most common causes of lymphocytosis. Lupus is a collagen vascular disease; HIV is a virus but actually causes a profound decrease in lymphocytes; and Hodgkin's is a lymphoma.

A–113

(C) Choice (A) are a type of ring found at the squamnocolumnar junction in the esophagus. Choice (B) describes a hiatus hernia, and choice (D) is descriptive of esophageal cancer.

Questions

Gastrointestinal

The highest levels of carcinoembryonic antigen (CEA) are typically seen in patients with

(A) diverticulitis
(B) pancreatic cancer
(C) cirrhosis
(D) colon cancer

Your Answer _____

Genitourinary

An elevated prostate-specific antigen (PSA) is non-specific, but a 30% increase in one year is more likely to indicate

(A) benign prostatic hypertrophy
(B) prostate cancer
(C) prostatitis
(D) cystitis

Your Answer _____

Correct Answers

A–114

(D) Colon cancer typically causes the highest elevation of CEA. However, elevated levels may be present in all the above conditions. The limitation of a CEA measurement is its poor sensitivity and specificity.

A–115

(B) PSA measurements must be interpreted in relationship to age and ethnicity, but a huge increase in a measurement trend likely indicates the presence of cancer. Further tests are usually necessary to confirm the diagnosis. A man with cystitis (choice D) should have no inherent change in PSA.

Questions

Hematology

You are checking laboratory reports from patients previously seen in your office. A WBC differential is reported as follows: Total WBC 11,000; 64.7% neutrophils; 23.3% lymphocytes; 7.2% monocytes; 2.8% eosinophils; and 0.6% basophils. Based on these results, you could assume that the patient has

(A) an infection
(B) a normal differential
(C) an allergic condition
(D) high levels of lead in the blood

Your Answer _____

_____

Gastrointestinal

Which of the following statements is/are true regarding Barrett's esophagus?

(A) It is a sequel of chronic alcohol ingestion.
(B) Columnar epithelium extends proximal to the gastro-esophageal junction.
(C) It is a sequel of chronic GERD.
(D) Both (B) and (C) are true.

Your Answer _____

_____

Correct Answers

A–116

(B) The numbers are within the range of normal. Total WBC level is slightly increased (normal is 4,500 to 10,000).

A–117

(D) Barrett's esophagus is a condition in which the esophagus changes so that some of its lining is replaced by a type of tissue (columnar) similar to that normally found in the intestine. It is associated with the very common condition of gastroesophageal reflux disease or GERD.

Questions

Q–118

Gastrointestinal

A patient presents with dysphagia and odynophagia; both are presenting symptoms in 60%–95% of patients with infectious esophagitis. The patient reports nausea, vomiting, diarrhea, fever, and weight loss as well. Which of the following agents is most likely the cause of this patient's condition?

(A) *Candida albicans*
(B) *Herpes simplex*
(C) Cytomegalovirus
(D) All of the above present with these symptoms.

Your Answer _____

Q–119

Endocrinology

Which of the following drugs would you NOT prescribe for a patient diagnosed with acute intermittent porphyria?

(A) Acetaminophen
(B) Glipizide
(C) Phenobarbital
(D) Temazepam

Your Answer _____

Correct Answers

A–118

(C) Cytomegalovirus (CMV) esophagitis often is only one component of a generalized CMV infection, which is consistent with this patient's report. In contrast, *Candida albicans* and *Herpes simplex* esophagitis usually are not associated with infection in other organs, and systemic symptoms are uncommon.

A–119

(C) Phenobarbital and other barbiturates have been implicated in acute attacks of porphyria. Other anticonvulsant drugs may also precipitate an attack. Acetaminophen, glipizide, and temazepam are safe to prescribe in patients with a history of porphyria.

Questions

Q–120

Gastroenterology

The term "backwash ileitis" refers to superficial inflammation of the most distal terminal ileum. This condition may be seen in patients with

(A) ulcerative colitis
(B) Crohn's disease
(C) diverticulitis
(D) salmonella infectious colitis

Your Answer _____

Q–121

Women's Health

Non-modifiable risk factors for breast cancer include all of the following EXCEPT

(A) increasing age
(B) hormone replacement therapy
(C) genetic inheritance
(D) early age at first menstruation

Your Answer _____

Correct Answers

A–120

(A) Ulcerative colitis, by definition, involves the colon. However, in patients who have chronic ulcerative colitis, the terminal ileum may show inflammatory and ulcerative changes also. It is termed "backwash ileitis" to distinguish it from involvement of the ileum in Crohn's disease.

A–121

(B) Increasing age is associated with a greater risk factor for breast cancer, and one cannot modify age. Neither can one's genetic makeup be modified; 5% to 10% of breast cancers are inherited as a result of gene mutation. Females beginning menstruation before the age of 12 and those who go through menopause after age 55 are at higher risk for breast cancer. These are non-modifiable risks. Use of estrogen plus progesterone replacement therapy after menopause increases the risk of breast cancer by 26% compared to the risk in women who have not used hormone replacement therapy. This, however, can be stopped; therefore this is a modifiable risk factor.

Questions

Gastroenterology

The most common cause of anal pain is

(A) a thrombosed external hemorrhoid
(B) an anal fissure
(C) an anorectal abscess
(D) *Herpes simplex* infection

Your Answer _____

Gastroenterology

Screening test(s) for Hepatitis B include immunoassays for

(A) HBeAg
(B) HBsAg
(C) anti-HBs
(D) both (B) and (C)

Your Answer _____

Correct Answers

A–122

(B) The most common cause of anal pain is an anal fissure. The second most common cause is a thrombosed external hemorrhoid; and the third most common is an anorectal abscess.

A–123

(D) Both hepatitis B surface antigen (HbsAg) and hepatitis B surface antibody (anti-HBs) are screening tests. Those who test positive for HBsAg will require further testing, including assays for HBeAg and others.

Questions

Q-124

Urology/Renal

Glycosuria is associated with all of the following EXCEPT

(A) diabetes mellitus
(B) urinary tract infection
(C) thiazide diuretics
(D) elevated glucose levels

Your Answer _____

Q-125

Pediatrics

The preferred site for a peripheral puncture on a newborn is the

(A) great toe
(B) earlobe
(C) lateral aspect of the heel
(D) abdominal subcutaneous tissue

Your Answer _____

Correct Answers

A–124

(B) Glycosuria is not associated with urinary tract infections.

A–125

(C) The newborn's heel contains the best capillary bed and is the preferred site for a peripheral puncture.

Questions

Q–126

Gastroenterology

Which of the characteristics listed below are more prominent in a patient with Crohn's disease?

(A) Smoker
(B) Rectal bleeding
(C) Diffuse, continuous superficial ulcerations
(D) Normal perianal findings

Your Answer _____

Q–127

Gastroenterology

Of the following treatment modalities, which one has shown little, if any, improvement in patients with ulcerative colitis?

(A) Cyclosporin
(B) Methotrexate
(C) Azothioprine
(D) Infliximab

Your Answer _____

Correct Answers

A–126

(A) The majority of patients with Crohn's disease will be smokers. The other three characteristics listed are more prominent in patients with ulcerative colitis. Interestingly, non-smokers are more at risk for ulcerative colitis than smokers, while the opposite is true for Crohn's disease.

A–127

(B) Despite early optimism, methotrexate has not been effective therapy for ulcerative colitis.

Questions

Hematology

Lab result		Normal value
Hgb	10.1 g/dL	12-15.5 g/dl
HCT	30%	35-45%
MCV	72 fL	80-100 fL
RDW	16	11.5-14.5
Reticulocyte Count	2.0%	0.5-2.5%

The above labs indicate:

(A) Iron deficiency
(B) Thalassemia
(C) Vitamin B$_{12}$ deficiency
(D) Hemolytic anemia

Your Answer _____

Women's Health

A 51-year-old female patient presents with a red, scaling, crusty patch that covers the nipple, areola, and surrounding skin. The lesion appears eczematous and is unilateral. You suspect a diagnosis of

(A) psoriasis
(B) Candida dermatitis
(C) Paget's disease of the breast
(D) inflammation of sebaceous glands in the areola

Your Answer _____

Correct Answers

A–128

(A) Anemia is classified as a Hgb/HCT of <12 g/dL/36% in women and 13 g/dL/41% in men. MCV describes the size of the RBC: microcytic is a MCV <77, macrocytic is a MCV >98 and normocytic is in between. RDW describes the variability of the RBC size, MCH describes the amount of hemoglobin in a RBC, and the reticulocyte count indicates increased destruction of, or a decreased production of, RBCs. This example shows a microcytic anemia with an elevated RDW and a normal reticulocyte count. Of all the choices, iron deficiency anemia is a microcytic anemia with an elevated RDW. Thalassemia also shows a microcytosis but has a normal RDW. B_{12} deficiency is a macrocytic anemia and a hemolytic anemia has an elevated reticulocyte count.

A–129

(C) The description is typical for surface manifestations of underlying ductal carcinoma. Psoriasis presents as well circumscribed silvery scaling plaques, but breast involvement is uncommon. Candida is more likely to occur in the skin folds under the breast. Sebaceous glands in the areola may become inflamed and, if so, will result in retention cysts that may become tender and suppurative.

Questions

General Medicine

When interviewing a patient of domestic violence, the interviewer uses the mnemonic HITS. The H stands for

(A) hit
(B) hurt
(C) hassle
(D) hinder

Your Answer _____

_____

EENT

A 14-year-old boy presents with a fever, sore throat, and right ear pain. The patient is drooling and his speech is muffled, a so-called "hot potato" voice. A CT scan shows the right tonsil to be displaced toward the midline. The most likely diagnosis is

(A) epiglotitis
(B) peritonsilar abscess
(C) streptococcal pharyngitis
(D) tonsillitis

Your Answer _____

_____

Correct Answers

A–130

(B) While all the choices will probably surface as descriptive of domestic violence, the H in the mnemonic HITS actually stands for "hurt."

A–131

(B) The description is classic for peritonsilar abscess, which is usually seen in adolescents and young adults. Epiglotitis is more common in children two to eight years of age. Patients also have drooling with this condition, but the problem involves the epiglottis, not the tonsils per se. In streptococcal pharnygitis, one sees tonsilar exudates, tender anterior adenopathy, and fever. Drooling is not a feature.

Questions

General Medicine

The ethics of medicine is based on four principles and as a health care provider you will be routinely faced with making ethical decisions, especially in caring for geriatric patients. One principle refers to the duty to do good for others, and specifically to avoid harm in the process. This principle is referred to as

(A) autonomy
(B) justice
(C) beneficence
(D) nonmaleficience

Your Answer _____

_____

Respiratory/EENT

A patient presents with symptoms consistent with sinusitis. Since only a small fraction of cases are bacterial in origin, you decide to treat this patient as if he has a viral sinusitis. All of the following treatment modalities are indicated EXCEPT

(A) analgesics
(B) topical heat
(C) decongestants
(D) antihistamines

Your Answer _____

_____

Correct Answers

A–132

(C) Beneficence means the act of doing good. Autonomy refers to one's right to control one's destiny. Justice focuses on nondiscrimination and the duty to treat individuals fairly, and nonmaleficience involves doing no harm and avoiding negligence that may lead to harm.

A–133

(D) Antihistamines can thicken secretions and impair drainage and are therefore contraindicated. Analgesics are appropriate to prescribe for pain relief; topical heat will provide comfort for the patient; and decongestants are the primary therapeutic modality as they promote drainage.

Questions

Neurology

A 28-year-old has been admitted to the hospital with a diagnosis of pancreatitis. On day three of the admission, he becomes acutely delirious. He is combative, tremulous, diaphoretic, and reports "seeing bugs" on his bed. What is the most likely diagnosis?

(A) Opiate intoxication
(B) Acute alcohol withdrawal
(C) Sepsis
(D) Acute paranoid schizophrenia

Your Answer _____

_____

Gastroenterology

The gold standard test for fecal fat analysis is the

(A) D-xylose absorption test
(B) bile acid breath test
(C) microscopic study of stool for increase in fat globules
(D) quantitative measurement of fecal fat

Your Answer _____

_____

Correct Answers

A–134

(B) The symptoms displayed by this patient are typical of acute alcohol withdrawal. His hospitalization with pancreatitis is also due to alcohol ingestion. With opiate intoxication, the patient would most likely be comatose with respiratory depression. If he were septic, he might have shaking chills, but a fever should also be present. Patients with acute paranoid schizophrenia may have visual hallucinations and may be combative, but there is no history to support this diagnosis.

A–135

(D) Stool is collected for three days and a quantitative measure of fecal fat performed. A D-xylose absorption test is done if the quantitative fecal fat is abnormal. The bile acid breath test is used for steatorrhea caused by suspected bacterial overgrowth. A microscopic study of stool is limited by the accuracy of the microscopist.

Questions

Radiology

Which of the following is NOT considered a nuclear medicine scan?

(A) HIDA study
(B) Colonic transit study
(C) Myocardial perfusion study
(D) Bone density study

Your Answer _____

Radiology

You need a chest X-ray that will provide the best possible view of the apices of the patient's lungs. You would order a

(A) frontal view or posterior-anterior (PA) view
(B) lateral view
(C) decubitus view
(D) lordotic view

Your Answer _____

Correct Answers

A–136

(D) A bone density study uses a very low level x-ray. This test should not be confused with a bone scan, which is a nuclear medicine test that involves a radioactive tracer being injected into the bone. The other studies are nuclear medicine scans.

A–137

(D) A lordotic view is used to visualize the apices of the lung. PA and lateral views are standard X-ray views and a decubitus view is useful for differentiating pleural effusions from consolidations.

Questions

General Medicine

You need to order IV fluids for your patient. The IV set delivers 15 drops/ml and you determine that the patient should receive 125 ml/hour. Your order will instruct the nurse to administer a 1000 ml bag of IV solution every

(A) 4 hours
(B) 6 hours
(C) 8 hours
(D) 12 hours

Your Answer _____

General Medicine/Genetics

The karyotype of an individual can be illustrated as a written expression. As such, a normal female and a normal male may be expressed by which written expression?

(A) 44, XX and 44, XY
(B) 46, XX and 46, XY
(C) 46, XXX and 46, XXY
(D) 44, XXY and 44, XYY

Your Answer _____

Correct Answers

A-138

(C) If the patient is to receive 125 ml/hour of fluid, it will take 8 hours to deliver 1000 ml.

A-139

(B) The correct expression for a normal female is 46 XX and for a normal male, 46 XY. Karyotype refers to the chromosomal makeup of an individual. There are 44 autosomes and 2 sex chromosomes in the human genome for a total of 46; 23 derived from each parent. The sex of an offspring is determined by the sex chromosome carried in the sperm.

Questions

Infectious Disease/Pediatrics

You see a baby that weighs 26 pounds. He has otitis media and you decide to treat him with 50 mg/kg/day of antibiotic suspension. The antibiotic is available in a concentration of 250 mg/5 ml. You want the mother to dose him every 8 hours. What dose will you prescribe?

(A) 50 mg
(B) 10 ml
(C) 4 ml
(D) 7.5 mg

Your Answer _____

Endocrinology

Insulin U-100 is manufactured in 10 ml vials. The concentration is

(A) 100 units/10 ml
(B) 10 ml/100 units
(C) 100 units/1 ml
(D) 10 units/10 ml

Your Answer _____

Correct Answers

A–140

(C) The mother would give the baby 4 ml of antibiotic suspension every 8 hours. 26 lbs/2.2 kg = 12 rounded up. 12 kg × 50 mg = 600/3 doses = 200 mg per dose. 200 mg/x ml = 250 mg/5 ml = 4 ml q 8 hours.

A–141

(C) U-100 means that for every 1 milliliter there are 100 units of insulin. This allows injections of very small quantities of fluid.

Questions

Endocrinology

The insulin with the longest duration of action is

(A) lispro
(B) regular
(C) NPH
(D) Levemir

Your Answer _____

General Medicine/Immunology

Skin testing can be done to identify the substances (allergens) that trigger an allergic reaction in a given patient. If a patient scheduled for skin testing were taking a second generation antihistamine, he should discontinue the drug how many days prior to the testing?

(A) 45–60 days
(B) 20–30 days
(C) 2–3 days
(D) 3–10 days

Your Answer _____

Correct Answers

A–142

(D) Levemir insulin has a duration of action of up to 24 hours. Lispro is a rapid acting insulin and has a duration of activity of 3–5 hours. Regular insulin is classified as short acting and lasts for 6–8 hours, and NPH has an intermediate range of activity of 18–20 hours.

A–143

(D) Antihistamines interfere with the development of the wheal and flare reaction and second generation antihistamines should be discontinued 3 to 10 days prior to skin testing. First-generation antihistamines may be stopped 2 to 3 days prior to testing.

Questions

Cardiovascular/Women's Health

All of the following are risk factors for cardiovascular disease in women EXCEPT

(A) a waist size of more than 35 inches
(B) triglyceride levels greater than 150 mg/dL
(C) HDL cholesterol greater than 50 mg/dL
(D) fasting blood glucose greater than 110 mg/dL

Your Answer _____

Cardiovascular

The "critical value" for triglycerides is

(A) > 500 mg/dL
(B) > 750 mg/dL
(C) > 1000 mg/dL
(D) > 5000 mg/dL

Your Answer _____

Correct Answers

A–144

(C) An HDL cholesterol ("good" cholesterol) less than 50 mg/dL is a risk factor along with the other three listed in the question.

A–145

(A) Triglycerides > 500 mg/dL will trigger a "critical value" report from the laboratory. A normal triglyceride is < 150 mg/dL and levels above 200 mg/dL are considered high. High levels *may* contribute to atherosclerosis, which increases the risk of stroke, heart attack, and heart disease. High levels are also often a sign of other conditions that increase the risk of heart disease and stroke, such as obesity and the metabolic syndrome or even poorly controlled diabetes. Levels > 1000 mg/dL present a substantial risk for pancreatitis, and levels > 5000 mg/dL puts the patient at risk for hepatospleenomegaly, corneal arcus, and other conditions.

Questions

Cardiovascular

Which of the following conditions is most likely to correlate with a triglyceride report of <49 mg/dL?

(A) Alcoholism
(B) Gout
(C) Hyperthyroidism
(D) Asthma

Your Answer _____

Cardiovascular

Homocysteine is derived from the breakdown of essential amino acids and if elevated >12mmol/L is an independent risk factor for heart and blood vessel disease. Certain drugs may elevate homocysteine levels. Elevated levels may be seen in patients taking

(A) metformin
(B) carbamazepine
(C) oral contraceptives
(D) all of the above

Your Answer _____

Correct Answers

A–146

(C) Hyperthyroidism and possibly some other autoimmune disorders may be associated with a lowering of triglycerides. Excessive alcohol ingestion is associated with an increase in triglycerides. Patient with gout also often have elevated triglyceride levels. There is no known direct correlation between asthma and hypotriglyceridemia.

A–147

(D) All of the drugs may elevate homocysteine to > 15 mmol/L which is in the dangerous zone.

Questions

General Medicine

In addition to being a risk factor for heart disease, elevated homocysteine levels have been associated with which of the following?

(A) Dementia
(B) Parkinson's disease
(C) Iron deficiency anemia
(D) Colon cancer

Your Answer _____

Dermatology

This condition is characterized by episodic, asymmetrical, non-pitting swelling of loose tissue, usually skin. It is usually nonerythematous and nonpruritic, and may be painless. It may persist for 24 hours or longer. Gastrointestinal involvement can cause crampy abdominal pain followed by watery diarrhea. This is descriptive of

(A) anaphylaxis
(B) dietary protein enterocolitis
(C) angioedema
(D) cutaneous porphyria

Your Answer _____

Correct Answers

A–148

(A) An association between elevated homocysteine levels and impaired cognitive function and dementia has been documented. Conversely, Parkinson's disease (PD) per se is not associated with elevated homocysteine levels but levodopa used in treating PD has been associated with elevation of homocysteine. Regarding choices (C) and (D), there is some evidence to suggest that folic acid deficiency (not iron) associated with hyperhomocysteinemia may increase the risk of developing colorectal cancer in patients who have inflammatory bowel disease.

A–149

(C) Angioedema is basically a cutaneous form of an allergic reaction. In a full anaphylactic reaction, there is an explosive release of inflammatory mediators into skin, the respiratory tract, and the circulatory system resulting in urticaria, wheezing, and hypotension. Dietary protein enterocolitis is most often seen in infants one to three months of age with intolerance to dietary protein. Patients will have recurrent vomiting and diarrhea. Cutaneous porphyria typically causes photosensitivity and blistering. It may be accompanied by itching, swelling, and increased hair growth on areas such as the forehead. Often, there is no abdominal pain, which distinguishes it from other porphyrias.

Questions

EENT

Complications of sinusitis may include which of the following?

(A) Cellulitis
(B) Cavernous sinus thrombosis
(C) Mucocele formation
(D) All of the above

Your Answer _____

Endocrinology

Which of the following statements related to glycosylated hemoglobin (HbA_{1c}) is true?

(A) It reflects the average blood glucose over the past two months.
(B) If a patient has had poor control of his/her diabetes, the test should be performed monthly.
(C) It is the primary test to monitor control of diabetic patients with acute renal failure.
(D) When elevated, there is a greater likelihood of heart failure after a myocardial infarction.

Your Answer _____

Correct Answers

A–150

(D) Choices (A), (B), and (C) are all complications of sinusitis; others include abscess formation and osteomyelitis. Appropriate treatment with antibiotics may prevent these complications.

A–151

(D) When glycosylated hemoglobin is elevated, there is a greater likelihood of heart failure following a myocardial infarction. The HbA_{1c} reflects the average blood glucose over the lifespan of a red blood cell, or 120 days. Therefore, the test should be done four times per year. Red blood cell survival is shortened in patients with chronic renal failure.

Questions

Pulmonary

SARS (severe acute respiratory syndrome) is usually caused by

(A) viruses
(B) *Streptococcus pneumonia*
(C) *Hemophilus influenza*
(D) mycoplasma

Your Answer _____

Pulmonary

Blood gas analyses gives information about a patient's

(A) acid-base balance
(B) metabolic status
(C) respiratory status
(D) All of the above

Your Answer _____

Correct Answers

A–152

(A)   Most cases of SARS are due to viruses. *Streptococcus pneumonia,* a bacterium, is the organism implicated in 30%–60% of cases of community acquired pneumonia. *Hemophilus influenza*, also a bacterium, is associated with many types of infections, both those acquired in and out of the hospital. Mycoplasma causes atypical pneumonia.

A–153

(D)   A blood gas analysis will provide information about the patient's acid-base balance, metabolic status, and respiratory status.

Questions

Pulmonary

You see a 40-year-old patient and order a blood gas analysis which reveals the following values: pH 7.5; HCO_3 31 mEq/L; $PaCO_2$ 48 mmHG. The patient has

(A) respiratory acidosis
(B) respiratory alkalosis
(C) metabolic acidosis
(D) metabolic alkalosis

Your Answer _____

_____

Hematology

One might see abnormal red blood cells described as "target cells" in a patient with

(A) mechanical heart valves
(B) sickle cell anemia
(C) a splenectomy
(D) Hodgkin's disease

Your Answer _____

_____

Correct Answers

(D) The patient has metabolic alkalosis. Normal blood gas values are: pH: 7.35–7.45; bicarbonate (HCO_3): 22–26 mEq/L; partial pressure of carbon dioxide ($PaCO_2$): 35–45 mmHg; partial pressure of oxygen (PaO_2): 75–100 mmHg. Vomiting is a common cause, but other causes, such as prolonged nasogastric suctioning, may also induce metabolic alkalosis. Respiratory acidosis may be seen in patients with obstructive lung disease. Hypoxemia may cause respiratory alkalosis. Patients with renal failure may have a metabolic acidosis.

(C) "Target cells" are RBCs characterized by a densely stained center surrounded by a pale, unstained ring. They are seen in patients who have had their spleen removed. Schistocytes are present in patients with mechanical heart valves, and crescent bodies are found in patients with sickle cell anemia. One sees lacunar histiocytes in Hodgkin's disease.

Questions

Hematology

A patient with renal disease will most often have which type of anemia?

(A) Normochromic
(B) Normocytic/hypochromic
(C) Microcytic/normochromic
(D) Macrocytic/normochromic

Your Answer _____

Infectious Disease

The Centers for Disease Control's (CDC's) campaign to prevent antimicrobial resistance in healthcare settings included all of the following EXCEPT

(A) vaccinations
(B) inserting catheters
(C) using local data
(D) breaking the chain of contagion

Your Answer _____

Correct Answers

A–156

(C) Patients with renal disease often exhibit a microcytic/normochromic anemia. A normochromic anemia is present in patients with acute blood loss or hemolytic anemia. Systemic disease or lead poisoning causes a microcytic/hypochromic anemia, and vitamin B12 or folate deficiency may lead to a macrocytic/normochromic anemia.

A–157

(B) All catheters should be removed from a patient as soon as medically feasible because catheters can be a source of bacterial contamination. Answers (A), (C), and (D) are recommendations of the CDC, as well as several others not listed.

Questions

Women's Health/Oncology

Which of the following tumor markers is used to detect or determine the extent of ovarian cancer?

(A) CA 19–9
(B) CA 27–29
(C) CA 15–3
(D) CA 125

Your Answer _____

Endocrine/Pharmacology

Which one of the following drugs causes elevation of thyroid stimulating hormone (TSH)?

(A) Amiodarone
(B) Aspirin
(C) Ketoconazole
(D) Prednisone

Your Answer _____

Correct Answers

A–158

(D) CA 125 will be elevated in more than 80% of females with ovarian cancer. CA 19–9 is a marker for pancreatic cancer. CA 27–29 and CA 15–3 are markers for breast cancer.

A–159

(A) Amiodarone will elevate TSH. The literature is inconsistent regarding the effects of aspirin. Some say that aspirin will decrease TSH, and others say there is no correlation. Ketoconazole does not affect the TSH level. Prednisone will decrease it.

Questions

Renal/Urology

Your first impression when you see RBC casts in a urine sample is that the patient has

(A) acute glomerulonephritis
(B) acute tubular nephrosis
(C) renal transplant rejection
(D) dehydration

Your Answer _____

Cardiovascular

You see a chronically ill patient who takes multiple drugs. In your follow-up care, you order serum electrolytes and learn that his sodium level is < 135 mEq/L. You suspect that this is drug related. Which of the following is most likely to cause hyponatremia?

(A) Calcium channel blockers
(B) Conjugated estrogens
(C) Laxatives
(D) ACE inhibitors

Your Answer _____

Correct Answers

A–160

(A) A patient with acute glomerulonephritis will have red cell casts in the urine. The presence of granular casts are a sign of underlying kidney disease but they are nonspecific and may be found in persons with chronic renal disease, acute tubular nephrosis, and renal transplant rejection. Hyaline casts may be present in normal individuals or in individuals who are dehydrated or participate in vigorous exercise or who are taking diuretic medicines.

A–161

(D) ACE inhibitors may induce hyponatremia. Estrogens and laxatives may cause hypernatremia; calcium channel blockers generally have no effect on sodium.

Questions

Pulmonary

Which of the following is not true regarding sarcoidosis?

(A) It is characterized by noncaseating granulomas in affected organs.

(B) Common symptoms include cough, dyspnea, and chest discomfort.

(C) It is responsive to corticosteroids.

(D) Angiotension-converting enzyme levels are used for diagnosis in addition to a tissue biopsy.

Your Answer _____

_____

Surgery

Which surgical procedure performed for purposes of sterilization can be reversed?

(A) Oophorectomy
(B) Tubal ligation
(C) Hysterectomy
(D) Orchiectomy

Your Answer _____

_____

Correct Answers

A–162

(D) Sarcoidosis is a multi-organ disease that predominately affects the lungs. It is characterized by noncaseating granulomas in affected organs including lungs, lymph nodes, eyes, skin, liver, spleen, and heart. Because it is predominantly found in the lungs, the most common symptoms are a dry cough, dyspnea, and chest discomfort. Ninety percent of cases are responsive to corticosteroids. Diagnosis is made by biopsy with histologic proof. Angiotensin-converting enzyme levels are followed as a marker for disease activity and not for diagnosis.

A–163

(B) A tubal ligation may be reversed, although there is no guarantee of fertility. All the other procedures are permanent and involve removal of organs.

Questions

Pulmonary

A fit, healthy person will probably have an oxygen saturation of

(A) 95–110 percent
(B) 80–90 percent
(C) 90–99 percent
(D) 100 percent

Your Answer _____

_____

Gastrointestinal/Genetics

Phenylketonuria is the most common of the enzyme abnormalities and it can be detected by the presence of excess amino acids in the urine. Which of the following characteristics is true about this disorder?

(A) It occurs in about 1:20,000 live births.
(B) It is an autosomal recessive inherited disorder.
(C) If not detected and treated early in life, it causes kidney failure.
(D) It is more common in African Americans than in Caucasians.

Your Answer _____

_____

Correct Answers

A–164

(C) Most fit, healthy people will have an oxygen saturation between 90–99%.

A–165

(A) PKU occurs in about 1 in 10,000 to 15,000 live births. It is of an autosomal recessive inheritance pattern and, when detected early and treated by diet low in phenyl-alamine, the patient can live a relatively normal life. It is more common in fair-skinned Caucasians.

Questions

Gastroenterology

A 33-year-old woman presents with symptoms that are variable and nonspecific, but include early satiety, anorexia, nausea, vomiting, and upper abdominal discomfort, including distention. The most likely diagnosis is

(A) functional dyspepsia
(B) GERD
(C) idiopathic gastroparesis
(D) partial gastric obstruction

Your Answer _____

_____

Psychology

Laxative abuse occurs regularly in certain groups of patients. Which one of the following is NOT one of those groups?

(A) Those with anorexia or bulimia nervosa
(B) Those who want to obtain a secondary gain from illness
(C) Those who want to poison themselves
(D) Those who want to escape from conflicts at home or at work

Your Answer _____

_____

Correct Answers

A–166

(C) These are classic symptoms for gastroparesis, a digestive disorder of abnormal or absent stomach motility. Functional dyspepsia has some symptoms in common with idiopathic gastroparesis, predominantly abdominal pain and discomfort. About one-third of patients with a diagnosis of functional dyspepsia will have delayed gastric emptying. GERD is characterized by burning esophageal pain.

A–167

(C) Persons who want to poison themselves will do so with a known poison or drug, such as ethylene glycol and acetaminophen. Anorexic or bulemic patients abuse laxatives as a way to help them maintain or lose weight. For some, the attention received from the induced illness is what is important for them while for others factitious diarrhea is a way of escape from conflicts at home or at work. For others, a psychological need to demonstrate a compassionate attitude is needed.

Questions

Gastroenterology

A patient presents with prolonged right upper quadrant (RUQ) pain and reports having a low grade fever. She also admits to anorexia, nausea, and vomiting. Which of the following physical examination findings is most predictive of acute cholecystitis?

(A)   A palpable gallbladder
(B)   RUQ pain
(C)   Generalized rebound tenderness
(D)   A positive Murphy's sign

Your Answer _____

Gastroenterology

Which of the following infectious diarrheas is/are transmitted person-to-person?

(A)   *Clostridium difficile*
(B)   *Giardia lamblia*
(C)   *Entomoeba histolytica*
(D)   All of the above

Your Answer _____

Correct Answers

A–168

(D) Murphy's sign is one of several maneuvers that may be helpful in diagnosing cholecystititis. It is a highly sensitive test but less specific and should not be depended upon to make the diagnosis, especially in the elderly. Generalized rebound tenderness is more suggestive of perforation and with acute appendicitis. RUQ pain could be present for many conditions.

A–169

(D) All of the organisms listed can be from person-to-person contamination.

Questions

Women's Health/Reproductive

According to the cervical cancer screening guidelines from the U.S. Preventive Services Task Force, 2012, all of the following are correct EXCEPT

(A) Women who have been vaccinated with 3 doses of the HPV vaccine should be screened the same as women who are unvaccinated with HPV.
(B) Women aged 30 to 65 should undergo screening with both cytologic exam and human papillomavirus testing every 5 years.
(C) Women who have had a supracervical hysterectomy for benign reasons no longer need cytological screening.
(D) Women older than 65 who have been adequately screened previously should not be screened.

Your Answer _____

Infectious Disease

Large outbreaks of hemorrhagic colitis have become common in the U.S. It occurs after ingestion of contaminated foods, such as hamburger meat. The organism responsible for the majority of these infections is

(A) *E. coli* 0157:H7
(B) Shigella species
(C) Cryptosporidium
(D) *Mycobacterium avium* complex

Your Answer _____

Correct Answers

A–170

(C) Women who have had a hysterectomy with removal of the cervix and no history of a high-grade pre-cancerous lesion or cervical cancer do not need cervical cancer screening. The woman in answer choice (C) still has a cervix and will need screening based on the screening guidelines. If low risk, women aged 21–35 should be screened every 3 years with cytology, and women ages 30-65 should be screened every 5 years with cytology and HPV typing. Administration of the HPV vaccine does not alter the cervical cancer screening guidelines.

A–171

(A) The causative microorganism in most instances is *E. coli* 0157:H7. Hemolytic uremic syndrome is a complication of the infection. Shigella organism can also cause early enteritis followed by colitis. Cryptosporidium is a parasite that contaminates water and causes epidemics of watery diarrhea. *Mycobacterium avium* complex is an opportunistic bacterium associated with diseases in immunocompromised patients.

Questions

Gastroenterology

The patient you are seeing has a history of short bowel syndrome secondary to extensive surgical resection. His diarrhea likely falls into which category?

(A) Watery
(B) Infectious
(C) Fatty
(D) Non-specific

Your Answer _____

Anatomy

Every tissue supplied by blood vessels has lymphatic vessels EXCEPT for the

(A) tongue and uterus
(B) placenta and brain
(C) omentum and adrenal gland
(D) eye and skin

Your Answer _____

Correct Answers

A–172

(C) This patient's diarrhea is probably due to fat malabsorption. Watery diarrhea results from osmotic changes due to drugs or secretory problems such as disordered bowel regulation, cancers, endocrine problems, or other diseases. Infectious diarrhea may be caused by viruses, bacteria, or parasites; and patients who have had surgical bowel resection may get these conditions but as the question is written it would not be the cause of this patient's diarrhea. Nonspecific diarrhea is often seen in young children (toddler's diarrhea) who have loose, watery stools without other symptoms. The child has a normal appetite and grows and develops normally. While no definitive cause is found, it often responds to a decrease in fluids, especially juice, for the toddler.

A–173

(B) Lymphatic vessels are essential in immunologic and metabolic processes. The only tissues not supplied with lymphatics are the placenta and the brain.

Questions

Gastrointestinal

Which of the following features suggest a diagnosis of irritable bowel syndrome?

(A) A history of diarrhea dated back to adolescence
(B) Exacerbation of symptoms with stress
(C) Passage of mucous
(D) All of the above

Your Answer _____

Women's Health

Primary amenorrhea is diagnosed by which of the following findings?

(A) Absence of menses with no evidence of breast development by age 14
(B) Absence of menses with breast development by age 16
(C) Absence of menses greater than 2 years after the onset of breast development
(D) All are true

Your Answer _____

Correct Answers

A–174

(D) All the listed symptoms occur with IBS.

A–175

(D) All of the choices are true and may describe primary amenorrhea.

Questions

General Medicine

Seventy-five percent of people in the U.S. have used at least one complementary or alternative medicine (CAM). Surveys have indicated that predictors of CAM use may include all but one of the following. Which one is NOT included?

(A) Female gender
(B) Caucasian race
(C) Lower socioeconomic status
(D) Higher levels of education

Your Answer _____

_____

Correct Answers

A–176

(C)   Persons of higher socioeconomic status are greater users of CAM. Many CAM users have chronic, non-life threatening medical conditions and may have an interest in spirituality. Some surveys also suggest very high usage in patients with cancer, HIV infection, fibromyalgia, and inflammatory bowel disease.

Questions

General Medicine

An unwary swimmer stepped on a buried stingray and received envenomation. Which of the following descriptions applies to injury from a stingray?

(A) An irritant dermatitis caused by the penetration of small spicules of calcium carbonate into the skin.

(B) An initial stinging sensation, paresthesia, and pruritis with local edema, blistering, and wheal formation.

(C) An intense pain initially which radiates up the affected limb. Pain is followed by an intense inflammatory reaction that can include erythema, edema, local hemorrhage, and tissue necrosis.

(D) Intense localized pain that peaks 30 to 60 minutes after the sting. The wound may become cyanotic and progress to necrosis.

Your Answer _____

_____

Correct Answers

A–177

(C) The stingray has a venomous spine near the base of the tail that creates a puncture wound when stepped on by the person. Release of the toxin can cause the signs and symptoms described in choice (C). Option (A) applies to an injury from sponges; option (B) from a jellyfish; and option (D) from a catfish.

Questions

General Medicine

Which of the following may be beneficial effects associated with fever in a person with a microbial infection?

(A) It decreases serum iron levels.
(B) It shifts metabolism away from glucose to fat and protein as energy sources.
(C) It actually kills microbes by virtue of the elevated heat.
(D) Both (A) and (B) are correct.

Your Answer _____

_____

General Medicine

Which of the following is/are necessary to define fever of unknown origin (FUO)?

(A) Duration of at least three weeks
(B) Temperature > 100.9°F on several occasions.
(C) Unable to make a diagnosis after at least three outpatient visits or three days in the hospital.
(D) All are necessary.

Your Answer _____

_____

Correct Answers

A–178

(D) Many microbes need iron for growth and it has been suggested that fever-induced hypoferremia is a helpful host defense mechanism. Glucose is an excellent substrate for bacteria and the shift of metabolism away from glucose may be helpful in eradicating the microbes. Option C is incorrect. Some bacteria are heat sensitive but body temperature does not get high enough to have this effect. Fever may, however, make it more difficult for the bacteria to function.

A–179

(D) All the responses are true. A fever of at least three weeks eliminates most short-lived fevers of microbial origin and most post-operative fevers. A temperature >100.9°F on several occasions eliminates people with prominent circadian fluctuations in body temperature. In the past, inpatient study was required to evaluate FUO, but with changing admission practices, intelligent and thorough study encompassing at least three outpatient visits or three days in the hospital is now considered sufficient.

Questions

Emergency Medicine

Parents bring their 11-year-old son to the emergency department. He experienced a sudden onset of severe unilateral scrotal pain in the absence of trauma. On physical examination you note the testis on the affected side is "high-riding and horizontally displaced" and that the cremasteric reflex is absent. The most likely diagnosis is

(A) testicular torsion
(B) appendiceal torsion
(C) epididymitis
(D) polyarteritis nodosa

Your Answer _____

_____

Cardiovascular

Which one of the following is an absolute contraindication to cardiac exercise testing?

(A) Left main coronary stenosis
(B) Unstable angina not previously stabilized with medical therapy
(C) Severe arterial hypertension
(D) High degree A–V block

Your Answer _____

_____

Correct Answers

A–180

(A) This is a classic presentation for testicular torsion. With appendiceal torsion, there is onset of subacute pain over several days and the cremasteric reflex is present. Epididymitis typically occurs in post-pubertal boys and men secondary to an infectious process. The cremasteric reflex will be present as well. Polyarteritis nodosa may cause testicular ischemia and infarction and is not specific to the testes. It is most common in men 40 to 50 years of age. It presents with fever, weight loss, and abdominal pain.

A–181

(B) Performing exercise testing in a person with unstable angina could cause the person to suffer a myocardial infarction and is an absolute contraindication to doing so. With any known cardiovascular disease, exercise testing should be performed under the supervision of a cardiologist. All other choices are relative contraindications to stress testing.

Questions

Emergency Medicine

Which of the following is/are descriptive of visceral pain?

(A)   It is primarily a response to distention and muscular contraction.

(B)   It is typically vague, dull, and nauseating.

(C)   It is poorly localized and tends to be referred to an area of embryonic origin.

(D)   All the above are descriptive of visceral pain.

Your Answer _____

_____

Emergency Medicine/Surgery

Of the following serious intra-abdominal disorders, all but one pose an immediate threat to life. Which one?

(A)   Perforated viscus

(B)   Severe acute pancreatitis

(C)   Mesenteric ischemia

(D)   Ruptured ectopic pregnancy

Your Answer _____

_____

Correct Answers

A–182

(D) All the responses are descriptive of visceral pain.

A–183

(B) All the conditions are serious and life threatening, but of those listed, severe acute pancreatitis poses the least emergency. The others require rapid diagnosis and surgery.

Questions

Emergency Medicine

Which description of abdominal pain best suits a diagnosis of intestinal obstruction?

(A) Severe pain in a patient who is lying still with a silent abdomen

(B) Colicky pain that becomes steady

(C) Tearing pain

(D) Waves of dull pain with vomiting

Your Answer _____

_____

Cardiovascular

All of the following are symptoms of aortic stenosis. Which symptom is indicative of the early stage of aortic stenosis?

(A) Exertional angina

(B) Decreased exercise tolerance

(C) There are no symptoms in the early stage.

(D) Dyspnea at rest

Your Answer _____

_____

Correct Answers

A–184

(C) Intestinal obstruction usually presents as waves of dull pain associated with vomiting because the intestinal contents cannot move distally. Choice (A) suggests peritonitis. Choice (B) suggests biliary colic, and choice (C) is descriptive of dissecting aneurysm.

A–185

(C) A patient with aortic stenosis is asymptomatic for a long period of time. The onset of symptoms depends on the age and physical conditioning of the patient. Symptoms begin during end-stage aortic stenosis and include: exertional angina, exertional dyspnea, or decreased exercise tolerance. Dyspnea at rest is not a recognized symptom of aortic stenosis.

Questions

Dermatology/Psychiatry

Trichotillomania is a form of nonscarring focal hair loss caused by

(A) a T-cell mediated autoimmune disorder
(B) compulsive hair pulling, twisting, or teasing
(C) primary hair shaft abnormalities
(D) a thyroid disorder

Your Answer _____

Emergency Medicine

A 37-year-old female patient is brought to the emergency department with complaints of severe, acute abdominal pain. On physical examination, you see ecchymoses around the umbilicus (Cullen's sign). While not diagnostic in and of itself, this finding could be caused by all of the following EXCEPT

(A) ruptured abdominal aortic aneurysm
(B) ruptured ectopic pregnancy
(C) hemorrhagic pancreatitis
(D) congestive hepatomegaly

Your Answer _____

Correct Answers

A–186

(B) Some patients with a compulsive disorder will pull out their hair leading to the condition called trichotillomania. Alopecia areata is caused by a T-cell disorder. Choices (C) and (D) cause nonscarring diffuse hair loss.

A–187

(D) Cullen's sign is an indication of intraperitoneal hemorrhage. Congestive hepatomegaly causes right upper quadrant pain along with an enlarged, tender liver.

Questions

Rheumatology/Musculoskeletal/
Laboratory Medicine

In an "acute phase" response, increases occur in all of the following EXCEPT

(A) C-reactive protein
(B) serum amyloid A protein
(C) prothrombin and fibrinogen
(D) serum albumin

Your Answer _____

Pediatrics

There are various ways to describe or classify newborn infants. One way is by birth weight. Which of the following signifies a normal birth weight?

(A) < 1000 grams
(B) 1000–1499 grams
(C) 1500–2499 grams
(D) ≥ 2500 grams

Your Answer _____

Correct Answers

A–188

(D) Albumin and transferring levels fall, accounting for the low serum iron and albumin levels that accompany inflammatory diseases. The C-reactive protein may increase 100 fold within 1–2 days. Not listed, the erythrocyte sedimentation rate, the time-honored test used to detect acute phase response, also increases.

A–189

(D) Newborn birth weight ≥ 2500 grams is considered normal. Infants weighing < 1000 grams are classified as extremely low birth weight. Those weighing 1000–1499 grams are classified as very low birth weight and those weighing 1500–2499 grams are low birth weight.

Questions

Pediatrics

Newborn infants may be classified by birth weight and gestational age. Which of the following classifies the infant as "weight small for gestational age?"

(A) Birth weight within the 10th and 90th percentiles on the intrauterine growth curve
(B) Birth weight < 10th percentile on the intrauterine growth curve
(C) Birth weight > 90th percentile on the intrauterine growth curve
(D) Infants are not classified in this way.

Your Answer _____

Neurology

Eliciting a 4+ reflex describes

(A) an average or normal response
(B) a brisker than average response but it is not necessarily indicative of disease
(C) a somewhat diminished reflex response
(D) a hyperactive reflex response

Your Answer _____

Correct Answers

A–190

(B) An infant whose birth weight is < 10th percentile on the intrauterine growth curve is classified as "weight small for gestational age (SGA)." An infant matching the description in (A) is classified as "weight appropriate for gestational age (AGA)." An infant matching description (C) is described as "weight large for gestational age (LGA)."

A–191

(D) A 4+ response is described as hyperactive. An average or normal response is labeled 2+. A 3+ response is brisker than average but not necessarily indicative of disease. A 1+ response is below normal.

Questions

Neurology

Clonus is synonymous with

(A) rhythmic oscillations between muscular contraction and relaxation
(B) infantile automatisms
(C) opisthotonus
(D) akathisia

Your Answer _____

_____

Dermatology/Immunology

The triple response of Lewis involves which combination listed below?

(A) Red line, flare around the line, wheal
(B) Bronchoconstriction, croup, rhinorrhea
(C) Cough, congestion, constipation
(D) Diarrhea, steatorrhea, right upper quadrant pain

Your Answer _____

_____

Correct Answers

A–192

(A) Clonus is a term that describes rhythmic oscillations between flexion and extension when eliciting reflexes. Infantile automatisms are reflexes present at birth or shortly after birth. Opisthotonus describes a body posture indicative of severe meningeal or brainstem irritation, and akathisia is restless pacing.

A–193

(A) These are the reactions that occur following firm stroking of the skin or injection of histamine into the skin. There is an initial red line due to capillary dilatation, followed by a flare with broadening erythema (arteriolar dilatation), and the formation of a wheal (fluid accumulation).

Questions

Dermatology

Firm stroking of the skin may elicit a wheal and erythema in 5% of a healthy population. This phenomenon is referred to as

(A) delayed pressure urticaria
(B) dermatographism
(C) vibratory urticaria
(D) geographism

Your Answer _____

Pediatrics

You are examining a newborn baby and notice an absence of the rooting reflex. This could signify

(A) that the baby is not hungry
(B) that the baby has a loss of perioral innervations
(C) severe generalized or central nervous system disease
(D) that the reflex is not present at birth but one that develops by one month of age

Your Answer _____

Correct Answers

A-194

(B) Dermatographism is a common finding in patients with idiopathic urticaria and is found in 5% of normal persons. A wheal and erythema will occur in the pattern applied to the skin. Delayed pressure urticaria may be seen in patients with urticaria who experience localized, continuous pressure. Vibratory urticaria follows massage and vigorous toweling. Geographism is a normal variant in the appearance of the human tongue.

A-195

(C) The rooting reflex should be present at birth as it helps the infant in breastfeeding. It disappears around three to four months of age as it gradually comes under voluntary control. To elicit the reflex, one strokes the infant's cheek or mouth and the baby will move its head in the direction of the stroke until the object is found.

Questions

Cardiovascular

You read in a patient's chart that he has pulsus paradoxus. This means that the

(A) pulse rate is < 60 beats/minute
(B) pulse is jerky with full expansion followed by sudden collapse
(C) amplitude of the pulse decreases on inspiration
(D) pulse amplitude increases when the patient is sitting or standing as compared with amplitude while supine

Your Answer _____

_____

EENT

The procedure that helps distinguish otitis externa from otitis media is

(A) pneumatic otoscopy
(B) needle aspiration
(C) movement of the external ear
(D) lateralization of sound to the affected ear

Your Answer _____

_____

Correct Answers

A–196

(C) Pulsus paradoxus is an abnormally large decrease in the pulse amplitude. A pulse rate < 60 beats/minute is described as bradycardia. A jerky pulse as described in choice (B) is called a Water-hammer pulse, and choice (D) is called a labile pulse.

A–197

(C) Pulling on the pinna will increase pain in otitis externa but not in otitis media, which has a deep-seated earache that interferes with activity or sleep. Pneumatic otoscopy evaluates the mobility or compliance of the tympanic membrane. A needle aspiration of fluid can be done to determine the cause of an inner-ear infection. Testing for lateralization of sound is a test of sensorineural hearing loss.

Questions

Psychiatry/General Medicine

Most organ systems suffer complications from well-established anorexia nervosa. Which one of the pairings below is NOT likely to happen?

(A) Heart—bradycardia and low blood pressure
(B) Intestines—diarrhea and abdominal pain
(C) Kidney—hypokalemia
(D) Musculoskeletal—decreased bone density

Your Answer _____

Women's Health/Reproductive

Which statement best defines herpes gestationis?

(A) It is an autoimmune disorder of pregnancy.
(B) The mother passes a primary herpetic infection to her fetus in utero.
(C) It is a benign dermatosis that usually arises late in the third trimester.
(D) It is a dark skin discoloration found on sun-exposed areas.

Your Answer _____

Correct Answers

A–198

(B) The most common gastrointestinal symptoms associated with anorexia nervosa are constipation and abdominal pain. As a result, patients frequently take large quantities of laxatives to help with weight loss. The other pairings are correct as written.

A–199

(A) Herpes gestationis is a rare autoimmune disorder of pregnancy. It is unrelated to the herpes virus infection but got its name because of the herpetiform blisters characteristic of herpes. A dark skin discoloration found on a pregnant woman in areas exposed to sun is called melasma.

Questions

Dermatology/Pediatrics

Ms. Jones gave birth to a baby girl one week ago and is very distraught that the baby now has a bright red growth on the bridge of her nose. The growth is diagnosed as a *strawberry hemangioma.* In counseling the mother, which one of the following would be appropriate?

(A) This type of hemangioma is harmless.
(B) It may continue to grow for about one year and then it will likely resolve on its on.
(C) The child will need surgery followed by chemotherapy as soon as arrangements can be made.
(D) Both (A) and (B) would be appropriate.

Your Answer _____

Dermatology

The most common atopic disorder in the United States is

(A) allergic conjunctivitis
(B) allergic asthma
(C) allergic rhinitis
(D) urticaria

Your Answer _____

Correct Answers

A–200

(D) Strawberry hemangiomas grow rapidly, particularly those near the eye. They are harmless growths located in the top layer of skin that may appear shortly after birth. They generally resolve on their own over time. The mother needs reassurance of this and also that the growth will be evaluated closely at every well-baby check-up.

A–201

(C) Allergic rhinitis is a collection of symptoms, primarily of the nose and eyes, caused by dust, pollen, or animal dander, in people who are allergic to these substances. It affects about 20% of the American population. Allergic conjunctivitis is closely related and shares the same causes and pathophysiology as allergic rhinitis. Asthma is a very common pediatric illness, and the incidence of allergic asthma is increasing. Urticaria is a prototypical manifestation of mast cell activation.

Questions

Gastrointestinal

What is the expected liver span when measured in the midclavicular line?

(A) <6 cm
(B) 6–12 cm
(C) 8–14 mm
(D) 12–16 cm

Your Answer _____

Gastrointestinal

Which of the following special clinical manifestations would NOT be useful in the diagnosis of appendicitis?

(A) Rovsing's sign
(B) Kehr's sign
(C) Iliopsoas sign
(D) Obturator sign

Your Answer _____

Correct Answers

A-202

(B) The usual span is approximately 6 to 12 cm when measured in the midclavicular line. A span greater than this may indicate liver enlargement, whereas a lesser span suggests atrophy.

A-203

(B) Kehr's sign is not used in the diagnosis of appendicitis. It is commonly associated with splenic rupture. This sign indicates a classic example of referred pain: irritation of the diaphragm is recognized by the phrenic nerve as pain in the area above the collarbone. All of the other signs are significant in diagnosing appendicitis.

Questions

Musculoskeletal

Leg pain in athletic individuals is usually caused by all of the following EXCEPT

(A) overuse injuries
(B) medial tibial stress syndrome
(C) transient synovitis
(D) stress fractures

Your Answer _____

Dermatology

All of the following are macular lesions EXCEPT

(A) cherry angiomas
(B) congenital nevi
(C) lentigines
(D) malignant melanomas

Your Answer _____

Correct Answers

A–204

(C) Transient synovitis is more commonly encountered in individuals who have had recent upper respiratory infections and is NOT necessarily related to activity.

A–205

(A) Cherry angiomas are described as papular lesions or dome-shaped elevations of the skin without visible fluid. The others are described as macular lesions or a change in skin color without elevation or depression.

Questions

Emergency Medicine/Radiology

A patient is brought to the emergency department following a fall in which he reportedly hit his head on the bathtub and became unconscious. Which of the following radiological test should be ordered first?

(A) Computed tomography (CT) without contrast
(B) MRI with I.V. contrast
(C) CT with contrast
(D) MRI without contrast

Your Answer _____

_____

Dermatology

Which of the following statements is/are true for kerato-acanthoma?

(A) It is a low-grade malignancy.
(B) It tends to occur in older individuals.
(C) It may be related to sun exposure.
(D) All are true statements.

Your Answer _____

_____

Correct Answers

A-206

(A) A CT without contrast is usually first in an emergency setting. It is excellent at identifying blood and is a fast exam that can be completed quickly. A CT with contrast could then be ordered if no abnormality is seen without contrast. Contrast will obscure an acute bleed.

A-207

(D) All of the statements are true. Keratocanthoma is a well differentiated squamous cell cancer.

Questions

HEENT/Mouth

A patient presents with painful vesicular eruptions of the lips and surrounding skin. In one area a small cluster of vesicles have broken and yellow-brown crusts have formed. The patient probably has

(A) chancre of syphilis
(B) actinic cheilitis
(C) carcinoma of the lip
(D) herpes simplex

Your Answer _____

Musculoskeletal/Rheumatology

A patient presents with monoarticular arthralgia. A complete history and physical examination reveals no significant trauma or focal bone pain, but an effusion and signs of inflammation are present. A joint fluid analysis revealed bone marrow elements. The diagnosis is most likely

(A) infectious arthritis
(B) intra-articular fracture
(C) bursitis
(D) pseudogout

Your Answer _____

Correct Answers

A–208

(D) This is a classic presentation for herpes simplex. A chancre presents as a firm, button-like lesion that ulcerates and may then become crusted. Actinic cheilitis presents as loss of redness of the lips along with scaling and thickness. Carcinoma is usually not painful.

A–209

(B) The presence of bone marrow elements points toward a fracture. With infectious arthritis, the joint fluid would contain elevated WBCs. Bursitis, by definition, is inflammation of a bursa so inflammatory signs/symptoms would be present, and with pseudogout (CPPD disease), crystals would be present.

Questions

Emergency Medicine

What is the No. 1 cause of accidental poisoning deaths in the United States?

(A) Acetaminophen overdose
(B) Tricyclic antidepressant overdose
(C) Carbon monoxide
(D) Acute alcohol intoxication

Your Answer _____

Musculoskeletal/Rheumatology

A patient gives a history of a slow but progressive poly-articular pain associated with mild joint stiffness, especially in the morning after awakening. Recently, mild joint swelling has also been noted. These symptoms suggest

(A) an inflammatory arthritis
(B) a non-inflammatory arthritis
(C) rheumatoid arthritis
(D) both (A) and (C) are possible

Your Answer _____

Correct Answers

A–210

(C) Accidental carbon monoxide poisoning is the leading cause of accidental poisoning deaths in the United States. It will show on a CT scan as symmetric, low attenuation changes in the globus pallidus. Choices (A) and (B) are drugs frequently used in intentional suicide attempts, and acute alcohol intoxication usually occurs in the context of partying.

A–211

(D) Joint pain, stiffness, and swelling even with joint rest are indicative of an inflammatory arthritis and help distinguish it from non-inflammatory arthritis.

Questions

Dermatology

Which one of the following skin disorders presents as smooth, pearl-colored lesions similar to very large comedones?

(A) Sebaceous hyperplasia
(B) Epidermal cysts
(C) Skin tags
(D) Verrucae

Your Answer _____

EENT/Ophthalmology

Which of the following statements is correct?

(A) Nystagmus present a few days after birth is normal.
(B) Alternating convergent strabismus persisting beyond four months of age may indicate ocular muscle weakness.
(C) Newborns with sub-conjunctival and sclera hemorrhages may have visual impairment.
(D) For the first three days of life, an infant's eyes remain fixed.

Your Answer _____

Correct Answers

A–212

(B) Comedones are small, flesh-colored bumps that are rough to the touch. They can be white or dark in color and are also known as acne. They result from plugged hair follicles. Epidermal cysts, also known as sebaceous cysts, present as smooth, pearl-colored, slow-growing benign lesions containing a collection of white, cheesy-like material. Sebaceous hyperplasia refers to enlarged sebaceous glands. Verrucae are warts, and skin tags are benign skin growths thought to be caused by skin friction.

A–213

(B) This is a true statement. Nystagmus present a few days after birth may indicate blindness. It is normal for newborns to have sub-conjunctival and/or sclera hemorrhages, and an infant's eyes may remain fixed for up to 10 days.

Questions

Musculoskeletal/Rheumatology

A boutonnière deformity describes

(A) hyperextension at the proximal interphalangeal joint
(B) hyperflexion at the distal interphalangeal joint
(C) hyperflexion at the proximal interphalangeal joint
(D) none of the above

Your Answer _____

HEENT/Ophthalmology

Detecting Brushfield's spots in the irises strongly suggests

(A) blindness
(B) Down syndrome
(C) Sjögren's syndrome
(D) sicca

Your Answer _____

Correct Answers

A–214

(D) A boutonnière deformity consists of hyperflexion at the proximal interphalangeal joint and hyperextension at the distal interphalangeal joint.

A–215

(B) Brushfield's spots refer to a speckled iris. They are little white spots that are slightly elevated on the surface of the iris arranged in a ring concentric with the pupil. These spots occur in normal children but are far more frequent in Down syndrome (trisomy 21). Sjögren's syndrome is an autoimmune disease in which the body's immune system mistakenly attacks its own moisture producing glands. The hallmark symptoms are dry eyes and dry mouth. Sicca is the term used to refer to the dry eyes and dry mouth of Sjögren's syndrome.

Questions

Musculoskeletal

Which of the following is NOT recognized as a clinical stage of gouty arthritis?

(A) Acute
(B) Primary
(C) Intercritical
(D) Chronic

Your Answer _____

Pediatrics

In addition to autistic disorder, which other disorder(s) falls under the umbrella of autistic spectrum disorders (ASDs)?

(A) Asperger's syndrome
(B) Rett syndrome
(C) Childhood disintegrative disorder
(D) All of the above fall under the category of ASD.

Your Answer _____

Correct Answers

A–216

(B) Gout is classified as either primary or secondary but once one has a diagnosis of gout, the stages are: acute, intercritical (time between attacks), and chronic or chronic tophaceous gout. Prior to the acute stage of gout, a patient may experience elevated uric acid levels and be considered to be in the asymptomatic stage of gouty arthritis.

A–217

(D) All the conditions listed fall under the category of autistic spectrum disorders. Asperger's is a milder variant of autism. Rett syndrome is a pervasive neurodevelopment disorder characterized by deceleration of head growth and small hands and feet. Children have symptoms of cognitive impairment and problems with socialization. Childhood disintegrative disorder occurs usually in three- to four-year-old children who were previously developing at a normal rate for age. With the onset of this disorder, children begin to deteriorate in language skills, socialization, and intellectual capacity.

Questions

Surgery/Pharmacology

Which of the following drug classes has been associated with causing osteonecrosis of the jaw?

(A) Triptans
(B) Statins
(C) Calcium channel blockers
(D) Bisphosphonates

Your Answer _____

_____

Cardiology

The preferred method for evaluation of patients with chest pain but with no known coronary artery disease is

(A) myocardial perfusion imaging
(B) electrocardiogram
(C) echocardiography
(D) cardiac catherization

Your Answer _____

_____

Correct Answers

A–218

(D) The use of bisphosphonates, especially IV adminis-tration of them, has been associated with osteonecrosis, primarily of the mandible, in people with predisposing factors such as dental disease, prior trauma, underlying carcinoma, or consumption of corticosteroids. The other medications listed have not been associated in any way with osteonecrosis of the jaw.

A–219

(A) Myocardial perfusion imaging helps determine whether the optimal therapy for a patient would be medical treatment or surgical intervention. It is often a follow-up to a regular stress test which yielded indeterminate results. An electrocardiogram is an examination that checks the electrical activity of the heart. Echocardiography uses sound waves to create a moving picture of the heart, and cardiac catherization is an invasive procedure to determine whether or not narrowing of the coronary arteries is pres-ent. However, cardiac catheterization is not the first proce-dure done to make that determination.

Questions

HEENT/Eyes

An elderly patient presents with inward turning of the lower lid lashes. His conjunctiva are irritated. The name of this condition is

(A) ptosis
(B) pinguecula
(C) entropion
(D) sty

Your Answer _____

Musculoskeletal/Rheumatology

All of the following statements regarding osteoarthritis are true EXCEPT that

(A) it is the most common arthritis
(B) it affects weight-bearing joints primarily
(C) chronically, it produces large joint effusions
(D) the primary risk factor is aging

Your Answer _____

Correct Answers

A–220

(C) Entropion is the condition of inward turning of the lower lid lashes. Ptosis refers to drooping of the eyelid. A pinguecula is a yellowish, somewhat triangular nodule in the bulbar conjuctiva. A sty is a painful infection around a hair follicle of the eyelashes.

A–221

(C) Osteoarthritis does not produce joint effusions, but rather wears away the cartilage. The other answers are correct.

Questions

HEENT/Mouth

A smooth and often sore tongue that has lost its papillae suggests a deficiency of

(A) niacin
(B) riboflavin
(C) iron pyridoxine
(D) any one of the above

Your Answer _____

Musculoskeletal/Rheumatology

A 36-year-old female presents with complaints of symmetrical erythema and edema of the small joints of her hands (PIPs and MCPs). She admits to morning stiffness, which takes an hour or so to improve after she arises. You order an erythrocyte sedimentation rate which is elevated and a rheumatoid factor (RF) which is negative. Which of the following is most likely given the above information?

(A) Osteoarthritis
(B) CREST syndrome
(C) Rheumatoid arthritis
(D) Ankylosing spondylitis

Your Answer _____

Correct Answers

A–222

(D) A deficiency of any one of the answer choices could result in a sore tongue with loss of papillae. Anticancer drugs can cause a similar condition.

A–223

(C) Rheumatoid arthritis is the most likely diagnosis because the patient has symmetrical joint involvement and prolonged morning stiffness. While a positive RF would have helped confirm the diagnosis, not all patients with rheumatoid arthritis will have a positive RF, especially early in the disease. Osteoarthritis typically involves weight-bearing joints and ankylosing spondylitis involves the sacroiliac joints and spinal column. CREST syndrome is used to describe limited scleroderma. CREST is the mnemonic for remembering the various components.

Questions

Dermatology

You note a papulosquamous eruption on a 16-year-old female. She described a single oval patch on her abdomen several days before the more generalized fawn-colored rash appeared. This rash is most prominent on her trunk and proximal upper and lower extremities. It is slightly itchy. The diagnosis is

(A) pityriasis rosea
(B) psoriasis
(C) atopic dermatitis
(D) tinea corporis

Your Answer _____

_____

Neurology

You are examining a patient for carpal tunnel syndrome and she has paresthesias located in all five digits. Paresthesia in which digits would be LEAST suggestive of median nerve neuropathy?

(A) first (thumb)
(B) third (long)
(C) fourth (ring)
(D) fifth (little)

Your Answer _____

_____

Correct Answers

A-224

(A) This is a classic presentation and history for pityriasis rosea. Skin lesions of psoriasis are red or pink areas of thickened, raised, and dry skin. Atopic dermatitis appears as red and flaky skin that is very itchy. Tinea corporis is a superficial fungal infection with a silvery scale that has the fine scale aong the leading edge.

A-225

(D) Carpal tunnel syndrome occurs when the median nerve, which runs from the forearm into the hand, becomes pressed or squeezed at the wrist. The median nerve controls sensations to the palm side of the thumb and fingers, although not the little finger.

Questions

Pulmonary

A 16-year-old male presents with a history of episodic wheezing, coughing, and dyspnea and is determined to have asthma by bronchoprovication spirometry. His symptoms occur most days of the week and with exercise, but rarely at night. What is the most appropriate therapy?

(A) Inhaled short-acting bronchodilator only
(B) Inhaled long-acting bronchodilator and inhaled corticosteroid
(C) Inhaled short-acting bronchodilator and oral corticosteroids
(D) Inhaled corticosteroids only

Your Answer _____

_____

Correct Answers

A–226

(B) According to the asthma treatment guidelines, this patient would be classified as having moderate, persistent asthma, aggravated by exercise. Suggested treatment for that classification is low-dose inhaled corticosteroids plus a long-acting bronchodilator. As each individual is different, the physician treating this patient could/would choose the most appropriate treatment based on the signs/symptoms/history of the patient.

Questions

Rheumatology

You see a 63-year-old woman who was recently diagnosed with temporal arteritis. She was prescribed corticosteroids and her headache improved. She comes today because she noticed a purplish discoloration around her eyes and she also admits to increasing difficulty arising from a sitting position. What is the most likely cause of both her discoloration and the weakness?

(A) There is probably no relation between the discoloration and the muscle weakness.

(B) These are consistent with dermatomyositis which can be associated with temporal arteritis.

(C) She probably has systemic lupus erythematosis.

(D) These are manifestations of polymyositis.

Your Answer _____

_____

Correct Answers

A–227

(B) Dermatomyositis (DM) is an idiopathic inflammatory myopathy (IIM) with characteristic cutaneous findings. Patients have a progressive proximal symmetrical muscle weakness. Cutaneous signs may include an intensely pruritic rash on exposed surfaces as well as a scaly scalp or diffuse hair loss. Systemic lupus erythematosis may also present with skin manifestations. However, the classic skin presentation is the presence of a butterfly rash on the face. Polymyositis is similar to dermatomyositis in terms of muscle weakness but unlike dermatomyositis, it does not involve the skin.

Questions

Endocrinology

Which of the following signs and symptoms do NOT describe hypothyroidism?

(A) Proximal muscle weakness
(B) Fatigue; lethargy
(C) Dry coarse skin
(D) Weight gain

Your Answer _____

Musculoskeletal/Rheumatology

You aspirate fluid from the knee of a middle-aged man who presents with knee pain, swelling, and warmth. Microscopic exam reveals needle-like crystals that are birefringent in polarized light. The birefringence is in the negative direction. The most likely explanation for the patient's knee pain is

(A) septic arthritis
(B) osteoarthritis
(C) psoriatic arthritis
(D) gouty arthritis

Your Answer _____

Correct Answers

A–228

(A) Proximal muscle weakness is commonly seen with hyperthyroidism; the other options are typical of hypothyroidism.

A–229

(D) Seeing birefringent crystals as described indicated sodium urate crystals and a diagnosis of gout. The other arthritides mentioned do not show crystals in the aspirate.

Questions

Rheumatology

Seronegative spondyloarthropathies have several findings in common. Which of the following is NOT a common finding?

(A) A negative rheumatoid factor
(B) Enthesitis and/or synovitis
(C) Symmetrical peripheral joint arthritis
(D) Onset in young adults

Your Answer _____

General Medicine

When working up a case of fever of unknown origin (FUO), what percentage of time will you find a cause for the fever?

(A) 10%
(B) 25%
(C) >75%
(D) Virtually always find a cause

Your Answer _____

Correct Answers

A–230

(C) Patients typically have asymmetrical peripheral joint arthritis. The other characteristics are present in seronegative spondyloarthropathies.

A–231

(C) FUOs are caused by infections (30–40%), neoplasms (20–30%), collagen vascular diseases (10–20%), and numerous miscellaneous diseases (15–20%). The literature also reveals that between 5 and 15% of FUO cases defy diagnosis, despite exhaustive studies.

Questions

Hematology

Warfarin differs from heparin in that it

(A) is administered subcutaneously
(B) has a delayed onset of action
(C) does not cross the placenta
(D) is not potentiated by the use of alcohol

Your Answer _____

_____

Cardiovascular

Which of the following compensatory mechanisms occur in heart failure?

(A) Increased sympathetic tone
(B) Salt and water retention
(C) Myocardial hypertrophy
(D) Both (A) and (B) occur

Your Answer _____

_____

Correct Answers

A–232

(B) Warfarin has a delayed onset of action because of the delay in Factor II (prothrombin) suppression. Heparin is administered concurrently with warfarin for four to five days to prevent thrombus propagation. Warfarin is given orally; heparin parenterally. Warfarin crosses the placenta and is a known teratogen; heparin does not in appreciable amounts. Alcohol consumption may interfere with how the liver metabolizes warfarin.

A–233

(D) Heart failure causes a decrease in cardiac output. The body attempts to compensate by vascular function (increasing blood pressure, heart rate, and contractility), blood volume (salt and water retention), and neurohumoral status (activating the RAAS). Myocardial hypertrophy is caused from chronic uncontrolled hypertension or heart valve stenosis.

Questions

Cardiovascular/Electrocardiology

Which antidysrhythmic drug binds to open sodium channels, prevents sodium influx, and treats supraventricular dysrhythmias?

(A) Lidocaine
(B) Quinidine
(C) Mexiletine
(D) Verapamil

Your Answer _____

_____

Musculoskeletal/Rheumatology

Which of the following orthopedic injuries has the highest likelihood of additional injuries elsewhere?

(A) Wrist scaphoid fracture
(B) Scapular fracture
(C) Hip dislocation
(D) Acromioclavicular joint dislocation

Your Answer _____

_____

Correct Answers

A–234

(B) Quinidine is a Class I antidysrhythmic agent that fits the description. Lidocaine and mexiletine are also sodium channel blockers but they have greater use in the management of ventricular dysrhythmias. Verapamil can be used to slow ventricular rate in patients with atrial fibrillation or atrial flutter, but it is a calcium channel blocker not a sodium channel blocker.

A–235

(B) Associated injuries are seen in up to 80–90% of patients with a scapular fracture. The associated injuries consist of other fractures, such as the clavicle, pulmonary injuries, brachial nerve injury, and shoulder dislocation.

Questions

Cardiovascular/Pharmacology

Toxicity from this drug is associated with corneal deposits, pulmonary fibrosis, and thyroid abnormalities.

(A) Dobutamine
(B) Disopyramide
(C) Amiodarone
(D) Propranolol

Your Answer _____

Dermatology

A 7-year-old school girl was taken to her family practitioner by her mother who was concerned about her daughter's itchy scalp. Other school children had similar symptoms over the past month. Based purely on the history available, the most likely diagnosis and treatment is

(A) Tinea capitis—Griseofulvin
(B) Scabies—Elimite Cream
(C) Pediculosis capitis—RID Shampoo
(D) Seborrhea—Selsun Blue Shampoo

Your Answer _____

Correct Answers

A–236

(C) Amiodarone is an antidysrhythmic agent used for various types of tachydysrhythmias. Unfortunately, it also has many side effects, which include those listed in the question.

A–237

(C) The most likely diagnosis is head lice and a common treatment is over-the-counter RID Shampoo. The other treatments are correctly matched with the diagnosis as well.

Questions

Neurology

Classic features of a migraine headache include:

(A) Unilateral periorbital stabbing headache that lasts for 30–90 minutes and occurs several times a day over weeks to months.

(B) A steady, bilateral band-like pain that occurs daily over a period of weeks to months.

(C) A throbbing, pulsatile pain that is unilateral, and is preceded by an aura.

(D) A sudden-onset, thunderclap headache.

Your Answer _____

_____

HEENT/Eyes

A funduscopic examination of a 62-year-old African American female shows a "copper-wire" appearance of arterioles. This patient probably has

(A) hypertension
(B) diabetes mellitus
(C) a subarachnoid hemorrhage
(D) methanol intoxication

Your Answer _____

_____

Correct Answers

A–238

(C) A migraine is a unilateral, throbbing pain on one side of the head preceded by an aura, and associated with photophobia, phonophobia, nausea, vomiting and/or neurologic signs. Migraine headaches are made worse with activity and last between 4 and 72 hours. A cluster headache is described as an "ice pick" stabbing through one's eye that persists for 15 to 180 minutes, and is usually followed by fatigue. It occurs in clusters several times a day for 2 weeks to 3 months, followed by a headache-free interval. A tension-type headache is a generalized pain involving the entire head or in a band-like pattern around the head. Tension-type headaches are not usually associated with nausea, vomiting, or photophobia, and are thought to be caused by increased muscle tension. A thunderclap headache is a severe headache that occurs suddenly and is caused by an intracranial bleed.

A–239

(A) Hypertension damages the small blood vessels in the retina, causing their walls to thicken and ultimately to decrease blood supply to the retina. Arteriolar narrowing due to thickening and opacification of arteriolar walls (copper wiring) may be seen in patients with long-standing hypertensive atherosclerosis. The changes seen in diabetic patients include venous engorgement, microaneurysms, and exudates. A patient with a subarachnoid hemorrhage will have blood in the center of the disc. The funduscopic examination of a patient with methanol intoxication will have a chocked disc with engorged veins.

Questions

Women's Health/Reproductive

A 38-year-old female presents to your clinic with amenor-rhea and dyspareunia. Her LMP was 12 months ago. On exam the vaginal mucosa lacks rugae and the cervix has small petechiae. Her serum TSH is 3.79 (normal range 0.5-5.0), her FSH is 61 (normal is <20), and a serum hCG is 0. Which of the following diagnoses best matches her clinical presentation?

(A) Premature ovarian failure
(B) Menopause transition
(C) Hypothyroidism
(D) Pregnancy

Your Answer _____

Gastrointestinal

Functional abdominal pain syndrome (FAPS) may be defined by which of the following?

(A) Pain that persists > 6 months without evidence of physiologic disease.
(B) Pain that shows no relationship to physiologic events (examples: meals, defecation, menses).
(C) Pain that interferes with daily functioning.
(D) All could define FAPS.

Your Answer _____

Correct Answers

A–240

(A) Premature ovarian failure (spontaneous primary ovarian insufficiency) is characterized by loss of menses, elevated FSH, and signs/symptoms of menopause such as vasomotor symptoms, vaginal atrophy, and amenorrhea. Menopause transition is the period leading up to menopause and may or may not have vaginal atrophy and an elevated FSH. Hypothyroidism would have an elevated TSH and hCG would be elevated in pregnancy.

A–241

(D) FAPS is poorly understood but seems to involve altered nociception. All the options listed could define FAPS.

Questions

Dermatology

Hair grows in cycles. Which cycle describes the short resting phase of hair growth?

(A) Anagen
(B) Telogen
(C) Catagen
(D) Exogen

Your Answer _____

_____

Infectious Disease

The term "black water fever" is associated with

(A) malaria
(B) plague
(C) tuberculosis
(D) amebiasis

Your Answer _____

_____

Correct Answers

A-242

(B) Telogen describes the resting phase of the hair follicle. At any given time, 10 to 15 percent of all hairs are in the telogen phase. Anagen describes the long growing phase; catagen, a brief apoptotic phase; and exogen describes the phase when hair falls out and a new one starts growing.

A-243

(A) Hemoglobinuria or "black water fever," due to massive intravascular hemolysis, can occur in patients with falciparum malaria. The urine darkens secondary to the released hemoglobin from the destruction of red blood cells.

Questions

Gastrointestinal

The "Rome Criteria" for diagnosis of irritable bowel syndrome (IBS) includes the presence of abdominal pain or discomfort for at least three days per month during the last three months, a change in consistency of stool, and which additional criterion?

(A) Improvement of pain with defecation
(B) Improvement of pain with antacids
(C) Onset of an episode associated with milk at mealtime
(D) Worsening of pain during menses

Your Answer _____

_____

HEENT/Eyes

Which statement correctly relates to the condition of non-paralytic strabismus?

(A) One or more of the eye muscles become paralyzed.
(B) Deviation varies depending on the direction of the gaze.
(C) It is caused by an imbalance in ocular muscle tone.
(D) It is characterized by a wide-eyed stare.

Your Answer _____

_____

Correct Answers

A–244

(A) A patient with IBS usually has an improvement of pain following a bowel movement. Option B is seen in patients with peptic ulcer disease. Option C is associated with patients who have lactose intolerance, and option D suggests endometriosis.

A–245

(C) Nonparalytic strabismus is caused by an imbalance in ocular muscle tone. One eye deviates from the other but each can move in all of the cardinal gaze directions. Options (A) and (B) are descriptive of paralytic strabismus. Option (D) describes a retracted lid.

Questions

Endocrinology

A patient presents with an elongated head with bony prominence of the forehead, nose, and lower jaw. Soft tissues of the nose, lips, and ears are also enlarged. Overall the facial features appear coarsened. These are suggestive of

(A) hypothyroidism
(B) nephrotic syndrome
(C) parotid gland enlargement
(D) acromegaly

Your Answer _____

Neurology

An oculomotor nerve palsy would cause

(A) anisocoria greater in dim light
(B) small, irregular pupils
(C) medial deviation of the affected eye
(D) a fixed pupil to light and near effort

Your Answer _____

Correct Answers

A–246

(D) Coarsening of facial features along with bony prominence of forehead, chin, and nose are seen in patients who have increased growth hormone excretion. Persons with acromegaly have this disorder. Persons with severe hypothyroidism may have dull, puffy facies (option A). A patient with nephrotic syndrome will have an edematous face with swelling around the eyes. A person with parotid gland enlargement will have swelling anterior to the ear lobes and above the angles of the jaw.

A–247

(D) The oculomotor nerve has a motor function that raises eyelids and participates in most extraocular movements. It also has a parasympathetic function that constricts the pupil and changes the shape of the lens. A nerve palsy would result in a fixed pupil to light and near effort. Anisocoria greater in dim light is caused by an interruption of sympathetic nerve supply. Small, irregular pupils are usually, but not always, caused by central nervous system syphilis. With an oculomotor nerve palsy, deviation of the eye would be laterally, not medially, if in fact there was deviation at all.

Questions

Emergency Medicine

A 14-year-old boy was hit in the left eye with a baseball. When examining him at the emergency room, you note that he tilts his head toward the affected eye and he states that he "sees double," especially when looking downward and inward with the left eye. His pupil is normal in size and reacts to light as expected. He has damaged cranial nerve

(A) II
(B) III
(C) IV
(D) VII

Your Answer _____

_____

Dermatology

A patient presents with angular cheilitis. Which one of the following is NOT a potential cause?

(A) Excessive exposure to sunlight
(B) Nutritional deficiency
(C) Overclosure of the mouth
(D) Yeast infection

Your Answer _____

_____

Correct Answers

A-248

(C) Damage to the trochlear nerve (IV) results in diplopia due to weakness of downward and inward eye movement. The patient compensates by tilting the head toward the affected side. The most common cause of this vertical diplopia is trauma to the orbit. Damage to cranial nerve II would be expected to convey some signs of visual loss and changes in the pupillary reaction to light. With damage to cranial nerve III, there should also be changes in the pupil. Cranial nerve VII, the facial nerve, is primarily a motor nerve that controls facial muscle movements.

A-249

(A) Excessive exposure to sunlight causes actinic cheilitis. Choices (B), (C), and (D) are all causes of angular cheilitis.

Questions

Geriatrics/Ophthalmology

The leading cause of vision loss in people over the age of 65 is

(A) glaucoma
(B) diabetic retinopathy
(C) macular degeneration
(D) eye injuries

Your Answer _____

HEENT/Mouth

A painful, small, round or oval ulcer that is white or yellowish gray surrounded by a halo of reddened mucosa typifies the common aphthous ulcer. These may occur in anyone but are more commonly seen in patients who

(A) chew tobacco
(B) have Crohn's disease
(C) have tori mandibularis
(D) have fissured tongue

Your Answer _____

Correct Answers

A–250

(C) Age-related macular degeneration accounts for 8,000,000 legally blind individuals worldwide. Glaucoma causes 5,000,000 cases of blindness worldwide, and eye injuries account for > 1,000,000 cases. Diabetic retinopathy is the leading cause of blindness among middle-aged Americans.

A–251

(B) Most patients with Crohn's disease have focal mucosal inflammation seen endoscopically and aphthous ulcers visible macroscopically. Patients who chew tobacco or use smokeless tobacco may present with changes of leukoplakia. Tori mandibularis is a bony growth in the mandible along the surface nearest to the tongue and is not associated with aphthous ulcers. Fissured tongue may occur with aging and is of little significance.

Questions

Dermatology/Genetics

A patient present with pigmented spots on the lips. The spots are more prominent than freckling of the surrounding skin. There is also pigment in the buccal mucosa. You diagnose Peutz-Jeghers syndrome. What associated condition will this patient likely have?

(A) Multiple intestinal polyps
(B) A seronegative spondyloarthropathy
(C) Uveitis
(D) Hereditary hemorrhagic telangiectasia

Your Answer _____

Pulmonary

Mesothelioma is a rare cancer caused by exposure to

(A) pesticides
(B) solvents
(C) ionizing radiation
(D) asbestos

Your Answer _____

Correct Answers

A–252

(A) Peutz-Jeghers syndrome is an autosomal dominant inherited disorder characterized by intestinal hamartomatous polyps in association with mucocutaneous melanocytic macules. Seronegative spondyloarthropathies are associated with joint disease and some also have uveitis. Hereditary hemorrhagic telangiectasia is present in an autosomal dominant genetic disorder known as Osler-Weber-Rendu syndrome.

A–253

(D) Mesothelioma is a form of cancer that is almost always caused by previous exposure to asbestos. Pesticides, solvents, and ionizing radiation are all associated with cancers in children.

Questions

HEENT/Ears

When performing the Weber test in a patient with unilateral conductive hearing loss, the sound will

(A) lateralize to the good ear
(B) lateralize to the impaired ear
(C) be better transmitted through bone than air (BC > AC)
(D) be better transmitted through air than through bone (AC > BC)

Your Answer _____

_____

Women's Health

Women having premenstrual disorders have significantly higher absenteeism from work and more ambulatory health care visits. Which of the following is a key consideration in diagnosing premenstrual disorders?

(A) Timing of symptoms
(B) Degree of self-medication
(C) Absence of endometriosis
(D) History of heavy menstrual flow

Your Answer _____

_____

Correct Answers

A–254

(B) The tuning fork is used to compare hearing by bone conduction with that by air conduction. With the Weber test, sound will lateralize to the impaired ear if the patient has a conductive hearing loss. It will lateralize to the unaffected ear if there is a sensorineural hearing loss. Bone conduction is assessed by using the Rinne test [options (C) and (D)].

A–255

(A) The timing of symptoms must be confined to the luteal phase of the menstrual cycle and resolve after the onset of menses.

Questions

Infectious Disease

A patient with HIV infection is susceptible to an opportunistic infection with *Pneumocystis jiroveci* when

(A) the CD_4^+ count falls below 200 cells/mm³
(B) the patient requires a protease inhibitor medication
(C) a resistance to an antiretroviral is demonstrated
(D) All of the above are present

Your Answer _____

_____

Pediatrics

A mother brings her four-year-old child to your clinic for a well-baby checkup. Upon examination of the child's ears, you note a large chalky white patch with irregular margins on the left tympanic membrane. Your notes in the child's chart would indicate

(A) perforation of the left eardrum
(B) serous effusion of the left ear
(C) tympanosclerosis of the left eardrum
(D) bullous myringitis of the left ear

Your Answer _____

_____

Correct Answers

A–256

(A) Opportunistic infections are by definition, opportunistic. In the patient with HIV infection, his/her immune system is generally able to resist infection with *Pneumocystis jiroveci* until the CD_4^+ count falls below 200 cells/mm^3. A protease inhibitor drug is often one in a combination of drugs prescribed at the beginning of drug therapy. Resistance may develop to an antiretroviral drug at a time when the patient's immune system is still relatively competent.

A–257

(C) The description (tympanosclerosis) is typical of an old episode of otitis media and is seldom clinically significant. Perforation would show as a hole in the left eardrum. If the child had a serous effusion, you would see amber colored fluid behind the eardrum. If the child had a bullous myringitis, he/she would not be well as this occurs with a bacterial or viral infection, and you would probably see a fretful child with hemorrhagic vesicles noted on the tympanic membrane.

Questions

Endocrinology

As a student, you are assigned to go to the eye clinic one day a week and perform funduscopic exams on all the patients who come for an appointment. In one elderly gentleman you describe your findings as: new blood vessels are present, which appear narrower than other blood vessels in the area and they form disorderly looking red arcades. When you look this up later, you discover that this patient probably has

(A) diabetes mellitus
(B) hypertension, uncontrolled
(C) acute traumatic brain injury
(D) changes consistent with normal aging

Your Answer _____

Women's Health

Which of the following therapies have FDA approval for treatment of premenstrual dysphoric disorder (PMDD)?

(A) Calcium carbonate
(B) Pyridoxine
(C) Spironolactone
(D) Drospirenone/ethinyl estradiol

Your Answer _____

Correct Answers

A–258

(A) The findings are consistent with the late proliferative stage of diabetes. With hypertension, focal or generalized narrowing of arterioles will be present along with abnormal arteriovenous crossings. A patient with a brain injury will often have a sudden increase in intracranial pressure and pre-retinal hemorrhage. There are no typical changes in the funduscopic examination related to aging except for the appearance of yellowish round spots in some people and blood vessels that appear straighter and narrower than in young people.

A–259

(D) Yaz, an oral contraceptive (drospirenone/ethinyl estradiol), has been proven to treat the emotional and physical symptoms of PMDD. It is derived from 17-alpha spironolactone and has antimineralocorticoid properties similar to spironolactone, which does not have FDA approval but is being studied for effectiveness in management of PMS and PMDD symptoms. Calcium supplementation has been associated with lower mean symptom complex scores and pyridoxine may be beneficial in doses < 100 mg/day, but they do not have FDA approval for this indication.

Questions

HEENT/Mouth

Which one of the following statements best describes Fordyce spots?

(A) Flat or mildly raised deep purple lesions located on the palate

(B) Thickened white patches that may occur anywhere on the oral mucosa

(C) Normal sebaceous glands that appear as small yellowish spots on the buccal mucosa or lips

(D) Small red spots that result when blood escapes from capillaries into tissues

Your Answer _____

Infectious Disease/Pharmacology

This antiretroviral drug is associated with CNS symptoms, such as insomnia and nightmares.

(A) Zidovudine
(B) Lamivudine
(C) Efavirenz
(D) Indinavir

Your Answer _____

Correct Answers

A–260

(C) Fordyce spots are normal sebaceous glands with a yellowish color. Option (A) is descriptive of Kaposi's sarcoma; option (B) of leukoplakia; and option (D) describes petechiae which appear subsequent to biting the jaw.

A–261

(C) Efavirenz is noted for causing CNS symptoms, especially insomnia and vivid nightmares. Zidovudine is associated with anemia and myopathy. Lamivudine is very well tolerated and indinavir may cause kidney stones.

Questions

HEENT/Mouth

Now relatively rare in the United States, a bluish-black discoloration of the gums at the margin of the teeth may signal chronic poisoning with

(A) mercury
(B) lithium
(C) lead
(D) aluminum

Your Answer _____

HEENT/Eyes/Anatomy

A 43-year-old patient states that he has lost the temporal half of each visual field. He is likely suffering from a lesion

(A) at the optic chiasm
(B) of the right optic nerve
(C) in the right optic tract
(D) in the right optic radiation

Your Answer _____

Correct Answers

A–262

(C) Lead poisoning results from chronic intoxication when lead is absorbed into the body. It commonly occurs in children when old, peeling lead paint is ingested; however, there are many other sources of potential contamination, including toys derived from foreign manufacturers. Symptoms may include colicky pains, muscular weakness or paralysis, and a dark line along the gums. Mercury is widely present in the environment. Fish often have high concentrations of mercury, and pregnant women who eat large quantities of fish may distribute the mercury compounds to the developing fetus, which may present with neurologic complications at birth. Lithium poisoning is also associated with neurological problems. Acute intoxication with aluminum is rare, but it may be seen in patients with kidney disease. It may cause anemia and there is speculation that toxicity may play a role in the development of Alzheimer's disease.

A–263

(A) A lesion of the optic chiasm causes a loss of vision in the temporal half of both visual fields: *bitemporal hemianopsia*. This kind of damage is most commonly caused by a tumor of the pituitary gland that compresses the chiasm. A lesion of the right optic nerve causes a total loss of vision in the right eye. A lesion of the right optic tract causes a complete loss of vision in the left hemifield: contralateral "homonymous" hemianopsia. A lesion of the right optic radiation also causes a loss of vision in the left hemifield.

Questions

Cardiovascular

"Red flags" that should raise suspicion for a diagnosis of a vasculitis syndrome include all of the following EXCEPT

(A) palpable purpura
(B) exematous lesions
(C) hemoptysis
(D) RBC casts in the urine

Your Answer _____

Musculoskeletal/Rheumatology

You have been following a 54-year-old female patient for several years who has Crohn's disease. She presents today with bilateral ankle erythema and states that she has had pain in the knees and ankles for several weeks. You suspect

(A) CPPD
(B) osteoarthritis
(C) reactive arthritis
(D) enteropathic arthritis

Your Answer _____

Correct Answers

A–264

(B) Lesions commonly seen in vasculitis syndromes include purpura, ulcers, livedo reticularis, or nodules. Dry exematous lesions are not typically a component of these syndromes. Palpable purpura is highly specific for small-vessel cutaneous vasculitis. RBC casts in the urine (glomerulonephritis) is a common cause of morbidity and mortality in Wegener granulomatosis, a relatively uncommon, potentially lethal disease of small and medium-sized vessels. Recurrent episodes of dyspnea, cough, chest pain, and hemoptysis are the primary clinical signs in Behcet's syndrome. Hemoptysis is also a finding in Wegener's granulomatosis.

A–265

(D) Enteropathic arthritis is the term used to capture conditions in which gut pathology is thought to be of pathogenic importance for developing joint disease. It is related to immunogenetic mechanisms. Calcium pyrophosphate dihydrate deposition disease (CPPD) is caused by deposition of the calcium crystals into the joint. Osteoarthritis is a degenerative arthritis, and reactive arthritis was formerly known as Reiter's disease and is caused by an infectious agent.

Questions

Cardiovascular

The most useful information to confirm Wegener granulomatosis (WG) is

(A) a laboratory request for c-ANCA
(B) presence of hemoptysis in the patient
(C) a chest X-ray
(D) a lung biopsy

Your Answer _____

Cardiovascular

The vasculitic syndrome associated with allergic rhinitis and significant eosinophilia is

(A) Churg-Strauss syndrome
(B) Kawasaki disease
(C) polyarteritis nodosa
(D) Wegener granulomatosis

Your Answer _____

Correct Answers

A–266

(A) If the entire clinical picture is compatible with WG and if alternative diagnoses have been ruled out, the finding of circulating cytoplasmic ANCA (c-ANCA) with anti-proteinase 3 specificity is sufficient to make the provisional diagnosis and initiate therapy.

A–267

(A) Churg-Strauss syndrome, or allergic granulomatosis angiitis, affects small to medium-sized arteries and veins. It occurs in patients with a history of atopy, asthma, or allergic rhinitis. Eosinophilia is characteristic and often of striking degree. In Wegener granulomatosis, eosinophilia may also be present but is more modest in its elevation. Differentiation between diseases can be done with a test for c-ANCA. Kawasaki disease causes dominant cutaneous and oral mucosal manifestations, fever, and coronary arteritis. Polyarteritis nodosa is a necrotization of medium-sized muscular arteries and is associated with peripheral neuropathy and bowel ischemia.

Questions

Cardiovascular

It is recommended to treat temporal/giant cell arteritis with high-dose steroids as soon as possible upon definitive diagnosis in order to prevent

(A) a cerebral vascular accident
(B) blindness
(C) a migraine headache
(D) tic douloureux

Your Answer _____

_____

Pulmonary

The pilocarpine iontophoresis "sweat test" is used to diagnose cystic fibrosis. Which statement about that test is true?

(A) Elevated sodium chloride levels (>50 mEq/L) are diagnostic in adults.
(B) A single test if elevated is sufficient for an accurate diagnosis.
(C) A normal test excludes the diagnosis.
(D) None are true.

Your Answer _____

_____

Correct Answers

A–268

(B) Giant cell arteritis is a systemic inflammatory arteritis of unknown etiology that affects medium- and large-sized arteries. One of the leading causes of morbidity is visual loss, which may progress to blindness in one or both eyes. Prompt treatment with high doses of corticosteroids usually relieves symptoms of arteritis and may prevent vision loss.

A–269

(D) None of the choices are true. A level > 80mEq/L is diagnostic in adults and two separate tests on consecutive days are required. Having a normal test does not exclude the diagnosis of cystic fibrosis.

Questions

Pulmonary

The most common type of bronchogenic carcinoma is

(A) small cell
(B) squamous cell
(C) adenocarcinoma
(D) large cell

Your Answer _____

General Medicine/Genetics

Which of the following statements regarding X-linked inheritance is/are true?

(A) There is no male-to-male transmission of the pheno-type.
(B) Disease incidence is greater in males than in females.
(C) All the daughters of an affected male are carriers.
(D) All are true statements.

Your Answer _____

Correct Answers

A–270

(C) Adenocarcinoma 40%; squamous cell 25–30%; small cell 10–15%; large cell 10–15%. Although the percentages are close, adenocarcinoma occurs more frequently than all the others.

A–271

(D) All the statements are true of X-linked inheritance.

Questions

Gastrointestinal

A 19-year-old woman presents with a history of intermittent abdominal pain of varying severity. She denies associated fever and reports complete recovery between attacks. In passing, she mentions mild numbness and tingling in both feet. You order a battery of laboratory tests and note the presence of hyponatremia. This history is suspicious for

(A) irritable bowel syndrome (IBS)
(B) acute intermittent porphyria
(C) alkaptonuria
(D) endometriosis

Your Answer _____

Women's Health/Pediatrics

You are working in an OB/GYN practice and review an ultrasound that shows increased nuchal thickness of the fetus. You notify the mother-to-be and ask her to come in for an alpha-fetoprotein test. You suspect the fetus may have

(A) Down syndrome
(B) homocystinuria
(C) Gaucher's disease
(D) Turner's syndrome

Your Answer _____

Correct Answers

A–272

(B) Acute intermittent porphyria is a metabolic disorder affecting the production of heme. It manifests itself by abdominal pain, neuropathies, and constipation. Irritable bowel syndrome typically manifests as episodes of both constipation and diarrhea with no lab abnormalities. Alkaptonuria is an inherited disorder characterized by degenerative disease that affects the spine and peripheral joints. Endometriosis is associated with severe pelvic pain, especially at the time of menses.

A–273

(A) Seeing increased nuchal thickness on an ultrasound is suspicious of a Down syndrome baby. Homocystinuria is a disorder whereby the body cannot process certain amino acids. It can be diagnosed by newborn screening. Patients become symptomatic in the third to fourth decades of life. Gaucher's disease is an inherited metabolic disorder in which high quantities of a fatty substance called glucocerebroside accumulate in various organs. Turner's syndrome is a chromosomal disorder affecting females that has several different manifestations. One characteristic is a webbed neck.

Questions

Emergency Medicine

The initial emergency management of a coma can be remembered by the mnemonic ABCD, for airway, breathing, circulation, and drugs. Three of the following four drugs should always be given. Which one of the following is NOT routinely administered?

(A) Dextrose
(B) Naloxone
(C) Flumazenil
(D) Thiamine

Your Answer _____

Emergency Medicine

A patient with a suspected poisoning is brought to the emergency department. You have no idea what the poisoning might be. Your physical examination reveals the following: bradycardia, miosis, sweating, hyperperistalsis, wheezing, drooling, and urinary incontinence. You know from the physical exam that the patient has a

(A) sympathomimetic syndrome
(B) sympatholytic syndrome
(C) cholinergic syndrome
(D) anticholinergic syndrome

Your Answer _____

Correct Answers

A–274

(C) Flumazenil is an antidote for benzodiazepine overdose. It should not be given if the patient has ingested a tricyclic antidepressant or has a seizure disorder. In the comatose patient, it is often impossible to know whether these conditions exist. Dextrose is routinely given to treat hypoglycemia, should it exist. Naloxone is an opioid antagonist given to reverse common drug overdoses. Thiamine is administered in those suspected of having marginal stores of thiamins, namely, alcoholics and malnourished patients.

A–275

(C) All the physical exam findings point to a parasympathomimetic response or cholinergic syndrome. Were it related to the sympathetic nervous system (sympathomimetic), the patient would be in a hyper-stimulant state. If it were sympatholytic, the patient would have a low blood pressure, slow pulse, decreased peristalsis, and small pupils. It is not an anticholinergic syndrome because the patient does not have tachycardia and increased body temperature, and no mention is made of flushed dry skin.

Questions

Pulmonary

You would expect to elicit all of the following signs in a person with a pleural effusion EXCEPT

(A) dullness to percussion
(B) egophony
(C) increased tactile fremitus
(D) distant breath sounds

Your Answer _____

_____

Pulmonary

All of the following are causes of respiratory alkalosis EXCEPT

(A) anxiety
(B) aspirin overdose
(C) severe pain
(D) opioid overdose

Your Answer _____

_____

Correct Answers

A–276

(C) You would expect decreased tactile fremitus, as well as the other signs listed.

A–277

(D) Excessive opioids can cause respiratory acidosis; all the others are associated with respiratory alkalosis.

Questions

Respiratory/Emergency Medicine

A 72-year-old woman with a history of congestive heart failure presents with increased shortness of breath and bilateral lower leg edema. Her ABGs are: pH 7.23; PO_2 52; PCO_2 60; HCO_3 27. What is her acid base disorder?

(A) Respiratory acidosis
(B) Respiratory alkalosis
(C) Metabolic acidosis
(D) Respiratory alkalosis

Your Answer _____

Respiratory

Complications associated with untreated sleep apnea include all of the following EXCEPT

(A) dysrhythmias
(B) intellectual deterioration
(C) hypotension
(D) anxiety

Your Answer _____

Correct Answers

A–278

(A) This woman has an acute respiratory acidosis based on the pH of 7.23 and an elevated pCO_2.

A–279

(C) Hypertension along with the other characteristics listed may be seen in patients with sleep apnea.

Questions

Renal/Urology

A 27-year-old man admits to painless scrotal swelling for the past 12–15 years. The swelling sometimes increases after exercise but then returns to its previous size. When asked, the patient does believe that the swelling is gradually increasing, but if so, it is very gradual. He denies additional symptoms. He is convinced that he has testicular cancer. Your physical exam confirmed the history and you noted no other abnormalities. The scrotal swelling transilluminated well. Your are pretty sure this man has a

(A) testicular tumor
(B) hernia
(C) orchitis
(D) hydrocele

Your Answer _____

_____

Correct Answers

A–280

(D) The history and physical exam are consistent with a hydrocele, which is a painless accumulation of fluid around a testicle. Testicular tumors can also cause a hydrocele, but the long history associated with this case makes this highly unlikely. A scrotal hernia is a complete inguinal hernia that is located in the scrotum. Orchitis is an acute inflammatory reaction of the testis secondary to an infection. It would not be painless.

Questions

Musculoskeletal/General Medicine

In a patient with Osgood-Schlatter's syndrome, you would expect to find which of the following?

(A) Tenderness of the tibial tuberosity
(B) A limp
(C) Pain on external rotation
(D) Point tenderness over the medial epicondyle of the elbow

Your Answer _____

Respiratory/General Medicine

All of the following statements are applicable to Pickwickian syndrome EXCEPT that

(A) patients have excessive daytime sleepiness
(B) patients have low oxygen blood levels
(C) it is worsened by calorie deprivation
(D) patients are at increased risk for accidents

Your Answer _____

Correct Answers

A–281

(A) Osgood-Schlatter's syndrome is seen in children and adolescents and involves pain and swelling of the tibia just below the kneecap. It is thought to be due to too much stress on the growing bones.

A–282

(C) Pickwickian syndrome is also known as obesity hypoventilation syndrome. It occurs in obese people in whom poor breathing leads to decreased oxygen blood levels and increased carbon dioxide levels. The patient has sleep apnea with resultant excessive daytime drowsiness. This leads to an increased incidence of accidents and errors in work performance. Treatment is directed at weight loss.

Questions

HEENT/Eyes

A 19-year-old presents with swelling between the left lower eyelid and the nose. She denies trauma, but admits to having seasonal allergies. She has mild tearing. Pressure produces regurgitation of material through the puncta. The diagnosis is

(A) sty
(B) dacryocystitis
(C) xanthelasma
(D) chalazion

Your Answer _____

_____

HEENT/Mouth

Torus palatinus is described as a

(A) smooth mass that juts down from the hard palate centrally.
(B) common variant of bony overgrowth at the palatine suture.
(C) carcinoma of bone
(D) Both (A) and (B) are descriptive of *torus palatinus.*

Your Answer _____

_____

Correct Answers

A-283

(B) Dacryocystitis is inflammation of the lacrimal sac, which fits the history given. A sty is inflammation around a hair follicle. Xanthelasma are raised, yellowish, well circumscribed plaques along the nasal portion of one or both eyes. A chalazion is a chronic inflammatory lesion involving the meibomian gland.

A-284

(D) *Torus palatinus* is a common, benign exostosis of bone of the hard palate. It is more common in women than men.

Questions

Hematology

Three of the four substances listed below can cause hemolysis in patients with glucose-6-phosphate dehydrogenase deficiency. Which one does NOT?

(A) Erythromycin
(B) Fava beans
(C) Sulfamethoxazole
(D) Chloroquin

Your Answer _____

Hematology

You see a patient who recently returned from Africa and who complains of nonspecific symptoms, including increased fatigue, shortness of breath, generalized weakness, dizziness, and palpitations. On physical examination you note jaundiced sclera and pallor in the palpebral conjunctiva and nail beds. The laboratory report shows a urine that is a reddish-brown in color, a high reticulocyte count and an elevated LDH. These findings indicate

(A) iron deficiency anemia
(B) hepatocullular jaundice
(C) active hemolysis
(D) a RBC membrane defect

Your Answer _____

Correct Answers

A–285

(A) Numerous substances, including choices (B), (C), and (D), may cause hemolysis if taken by a person with G-6-PD deficiency. Erythromycin is not known to cause such a problem.

A–286

(C) Active hemolysis is the correct choice. In iron deficiency anemia, a patient could feel fatigued, breathless, and dizzy and have generalized weakness due to the diminished oxygen content in the blood. However, icterus and discoloration of the urine would be absent. Hepatocellular jaundice is usually caused by infections, drugs, alcohol abuse, etc., which does not fit the history of this patient. An RBC membrane defect causes a hereditary form of hemolytic anemia. An RBC evaluation will show abnormalities in the shape of the cells. This was not mentioned in the patient's symptoms.

Questions

Hematology

A normal red blood cell has a life span of

(A) 40 days
(B) 70 days
(C) 120 days
(D) 180 days

Your Answer _____

_____

Renal

Patients receiving chronic dialysis treatments are considered to have chronic kidney disease (CKD) stage

(A) 2
(B) 3
(C) 4
(D) 5

Your Answer _____

_____

Correct Answers

A–287

(C) The average life span of a normal RBC is 120 days.

A–288

(D) Patients on chronic dialysis are considered CKD Stage 5. The National Kidney Foundation created a guideline to help identify each level of kidney disease. The glomerular filtration rate (GFR) is the number used to classify a person's stage of kidney disease. Stage 2 is mild CKD (GFR 60–89 ml/min); Stage 3 is moderate CKD (GFR 30–59 ml/min); and Stage 4 is severe CKD (GFR 15–29 ml/min). Stage 5 is end stage CKD (less than GFR 15 ml/min).

Questions

Respiratory

You see a patient with asthma who tells you that he has symptoms every day and more than one night per week. His PEF average is 60–80% of his personal best peak flow. His asthma would be classified as

(A) mild intermittent
(B) mild persistent
(C) moderate persistent
(D) severe persistent

Your Answer _____

Respiratory

Patients with emphysema are commonly referred to as *pink puffers*. They have all the following characteristics EXCEPT that they

(A) are generally thin
(B) are pale
(C) have pursed-lip breathing
(D) have tachypnea

Your Answer _____

Correct Answers

A–289

(C) This patient has persistent asthma, and the fact that he has symptoms on a daily basis classifies it as moderately severe. The mild-intermittent classification has symptoms ≤2/week and nighttime symptoms ≤2 nights/month. In mild persistent asthma, symptoms are present at >2/week and > 2 nights/month. The patient with severe persistent asthma has symptoms continually during the day and frequently at night.

A–290

(B) Patients with emphysema have a flushed appearance, providing the "pink" description in the nickname, along with the other characteristics.

Questions

Respiratory

Patients with chronic bronchitis are referred to as *blue boaters.* They have the following characteristics EXCEPT for

(A) chronic mucous production
(B) cyanosis
(C) peripheral edema
(D) underweight

Your Answer _____

Respiratory

A patient is brought to the emergency department with a sudden onset of shortness of breath, along with chest pain that increases with breathing and coughing. The cough produces blood-tinged sputum. He also complains of left leg pain. The diagnosis is

(A) pulmonary embolism
(B) acute myocardial infarction
(C) bleeding gastric ulcer
(D) pulmonary infiltrate, probably bacterial

Your Answer _____

Correct Answers

A–291

(D) *Blue boaters* tend to be overweight and have the other characteristics; plus, they may have right ventricular failure and pulmonary hypertension.

A–292

(A) The patient history is consistent with a pulmonary embolism. Acute MI causes a crushing type of chest pain that doesn't vary with breathing. A bacterial infection would not present with a sudden onset of chest pain and the history is not consistent with a GI problem.

Questions

Pediatrics

In your examination of a male child, who you suspect of having an autistic spectrum disorder, you note a long face and prominent ears. You would want to rule out which disorder?

(A) Tuberous sclerosis
(B) Rett's disorder
(C) Fragile X syndrome
(D) Down syndrome

Your Answer _____

_____

HEENT/Eyes

Which statement is TRUE for people having astigmatism?

(A) They usually have eyeballs that are too large for their lens and cornea to focus light properly on their retina.
(B) They have eyeballs that are too small for the lens and cornea to focus light properly on the retina.
(C) They have irregularly shaped corneas.
(D) They have increased intraocular pressure which damages the optic nerve.

Your Answer _____

_____

Correct Answers

A–293

(C) Fragile X syndrome is the most common known cause of autism or "autistic like behaviors." It has the features mentioned in the other choices, especially prominent after age ten, plus others, including atypical social development, particularly shyness. Tuberous sclerosis is a rare genetic disease that causes benign tumors to grow in the brain and on other vital organs. It also has other symptoms such a seizures, mental retardation, and behavioral disorders. Rett's disorder is included in the classification of a Pervasive Developmental Disorder and may be confused early with autism. Profound mental retardation is usually present. Down syndrome children have a characteristic physical phenotype (unlike FXS), as well as diminished cognitive abilities.

A–294

(C) Persons with astigmatism have irregularly shaped corneas. Option (A) is true for myopia; option (B) is true for hyperopia; and option (D) refers to glaucoma.

Questions

Hematology

Burkitt's lymphoma is a very fast growing form of non-Hodgkin's lymphoma. Which of the following statements is FALSE regarding this lymphoma?

(A) In the more common type seen in the United States, it usually starts in the abdomen.
(B) It is more common in females than males.
(C) It causes rapid growth of the lymph nodes.
(D) More than half of the patients can be cured with intensive chemotherapy.

Your Answer _____

_____

Correct Answers

A–295

(B) Burkitt's lymphoma is more commonly seen in males, not females. The other statements are true.

Questions

Dermatology

A 9-year-old female presents with an erythematous, scaly rash on the scalp, side of the nose, and behind her ears. The rash has been present for 6 months and various OTC lotions, creams, and shampoos have not been effective. She has a history of seasonal allergies which are well controlled with an OTC antihistamine. She has not used any new shampoos or soaps. What is the best treatment?

(A) Pimecrolimus applied topically
(B) Ketoconazole by mouth
(C) Ketoconazole applied topically
(D) Mupirocin applied topically

Your Answer _____

Dermatology

Syringomas are

(A) benign sweat gland tumors that are generally confined to the eyelids
(B) hyperplastic sebaceous glands
(C) discrete white papules that appear as small, closed comedones
(D) patulous follicles that look like warts

Your Answer _____

Correct Answers

(C) The dermatitis described in this clinical scenario is in a very typical description of seborrheic dermatitis. Seborrheic dermatitis is found in areas with sebaceous glands such as the scalp, face, and intertriginous areas. Ketoconazole, used topically, is an effective treatment. Pimecrolimus is a topical calcineurin inhibitor and blocks inflammation but is not approved to treat seborrhea. Mupirocin is a topical antibiotic will not be effective in treating seborrheic dermatitis. Ketoconazole orally is not necessary for seborrhea of the face.

(A) Syringomas are harmless sweat gland tumors typically clustered on eyelids. Sebaceous hyperplasia is a common, benign condition of sebaceous glands in older adults. The papules are seen on the nose, cheeks, and forehead for the most part. Option (C) is descriptive of milia. Seborrheic keratosis [Option (D)] are sometimes referred to as barnacles because of their "stuck on" appearance on the skin. They arise from the epidermis but do not extend deep into the skin like warts.

Questions

HEENT/Eyes

A patient complains of moderately aching deep pain in the left eye and claims some visual loss. Pain is worse when exposed to bright light. Physical examination reveals erythema, a small pupil and slight cloudiness of the left cornea. There is no ocular discharge. Which of the following choices is the most likely diagnosis?

(A) Acute conjunctivitis
(B) Acute angle closure glaucoma
(C) Acute iritis
(D) Corneal infection

Your Answer _____

Musculoskeletal/Radiology

You review an X-ray of the lateral lumbar spine and note anterior displacement of the vertebra at the L5-S1 location. The name for this condition is

(A) spondylolysis
(B) herniated disc
(C) spondyloarthritis
(D) spondylolithesis

Your Answer _____

Correct Answers

A–298

(C) Acute iritis or anterior uveitis is the most likely diagnosis. Acute angle closure glaucoma is relatively rare and presents with severe, aching deep pain with decreased vision, headache, halos around lights, fixed, mid-dilated pupils, red eyes, nausea, and vomiting. Acute conjunctivitis causes mild discomfort and a watery or mucopurulent discharge. A corneal infection produces moderately severe superficial pain with a watery or purulent discharge.

A–299

(D) Spondylolithesis is the name used to describe the anterior displacement of a vertebra or the vertebral column in relation to the vertebrae below. Spondylolysis is a specific defect in the connection between vertebrae. This defect can lead to stress fractures in the vertebrae that, over time, allows one vertebrae to slip out of place or lead to spondylolithesis. A herniated disc occurs when part of the center nucleus pushes through the outer edge of the disk and back toward the spinal canal. Spondyloarthritis is a classification that houses a family of inflammatory arthritic problems.

Questions

Neurology

Most neural tube defects (NTDs) can be detected during pregnancy by which of the following prenatal tests?

(A) maternal serum alpha-fetoprotein
(B) High resolution ultrasound
(C) Amniocentesis
(D) Any one of these tests may detect a NTD.

Your Answer _____

_____

EENT

A patient presents with a complaint of dizziness. Questioning from you reveals that the patient is experiencing brief episodes of mild to intense dizziness associated with specific changes with the positioning of her head. She is otherwise without complaints. She is experiencing

(A) Ménierè's disease
(B) acute otitis media
(C) benign paroxysmal positional vertigo
(D) Cogan's syndrome

Your Answer _____

_____

Correct Answers

A–300

(D) Any of the tests can be used. The maternal serum alpha-fetoprotein test is performed on the pregnant woman's blood at 16 to 18 weeks of pregnancy. High resolution ultrasound may detect a defect visually after 18 weeks of pregnancy. Amniocentesis is effective after 15 weeks of pregnancy.

A–301

(C) Benign paroxysmal positional vertigo is brought on by particular changes in head position and lasts for only a few seconds. Ménierè's disease is characterized by episodes (typically lasting for hours) of ear pressure, roaring in the ears and decreased hearing, along with vertigo. Acute otitis media is accompanied more by ear pain but a person may experience some vertigo. Cogan's syndrome, which is thought to be an autoimmune disease, is characterized by dizziness, hearing loss, and interstitial keratitis.

Questions

Gastrointestinal

Acute pancreatitis can be caused by all of the following EXCEPT

(A) Chronic alcohol use
(B) Triglycerides elevated to greater than 500.
(C) Choledocolithiasis
(D) Endoscopic retrograde cholangiopancreatography (ERCP).

Your Answer _____

Correct Answers

A-302

(B) Risk factors for acute pancreatitis include: pancreas divisum, sphincter of Oddi dysfunction, autoimmune diseases, common bile duct stones, chronic alcohol use, hypercalcemia, infections, pancreatic tumors, post-procedure ERCP, trauma, and hypertriglyceridemia. Although triglycerides greater than 500 are a significant abnormality, triglycerides above 1,000 are a risk factor for pancreatitis.

Questions

Emergency Medicine

You are taking weekend calls and receive a call from a 17-year-old male who says that while playing football, he failed to make a clean catch and "jammed" his right index finger. He is in considerable pain and reports mild swelling but can make a fist. Appropriate management is to tell the patient

(A) that he has a mild sprain and to wrap the hand with an ACE bandage.

(B) to take aspirin and if he feels comfortable enough to continue playing football.

(C) to tape the finger to an adjoining finger and continue playing if it feels okay.

(D) to tape the finger to an adjoining finger and go to the emergency room for evaluation.

Your Answer _____

_____

Correct Answers

A–303

(D) A jammed finger can be painful and may need no more than splinting, but since this patient has swelling, it should be evaluated by a medical professional to rule out fracture. It is unlikely that the finger is dislocated based on the history. The ultimate treatment may be to simply instruct the patient to use warm soaks in Epsom salt bath for relief followed by taping the injured finger to an adjoining finger. Simple over-the-counter analgesic for a few days may also be recommended.

Questions

Hematology

A 44-year-old man has had a weeklong course of fever and mental confusion. Physical examination shows T 100.8°F, P 99/minute, RR 20/minute, and BP 102/60 mmHg. He has widespread petechiae on mucosal surfaces and skin. Laboratory studies show a BUN of 50 mg/dL and creatinine 5.3 mg/dL. His hemoglobin is 12.4 g/dL, hematocrit 37.2%, MCV 94 fL, platelet count 19,200/mm³, and WBC count 8200/mm³. Schistocytes are seen on his peripheral blood smear. He is given a platelet transfusion but continues to deteriorate and dies. At autopsy, pink hyaline thrombi are found in small myocardial arteries. Which of the following is the most likely diagnosis?

(A) Disseminated intravascular coagulation (DIC)
(B) Warm autoimmune hemolytic anemia
(C) Thrombotic thrombocytopenic purpura (TTP)
(D) Trousseau Syndrome

Your Answer _____

_____

Correct Answers

A–304

(C) TTP is most likely due to the hyaline thrombi. TTP can lead to low platelets, abnormal kidney function, and problems with the nervous system. Most cases have no known cause. Typical symptoms may include fever, pallor, heart rate >100 beats/min, confusion, changes in consciousness, and bleeding into the skin and mucous membranes.

Questions

Neurology

A Babinski reflex is a test for dysfunction of

(A) the corticospinal tract
(B) cranial nerve 12
(C) the medial clunial nerves
(D) sacral nerve 5

Your Answer _____

Psychiatry

This condition is marked by compulsive substance use that is coupled with episodes of substance craving. The condition is termed

(A) tolerance
(B) abuse
(C) dependency
(D) obsession

Your Answer _____

Correct Answers

A–305

(A) A Babinski's reflex tests for dysfunction in a part of the central nervous system called the pyramidal tract or corticospinal tract. Cranial nerve 12 provides motor innervation to the glossal muscles. The medial clunial nerves innervate the skin of the buttocks. Sacral nerve 5 supplies the coccygeus muscle.

A–306

(C) Dependency is a term that is synonymous with the old term "addiction" in which the habitual use of a substance creates a state whereby negative physical symptoms occur if the substance is not ingested on a fixed schedule. As addiction progresses, increasingly more of the substance of abuse is needed to produce the reward in the brain. This is called tolerance and it drives addicts to use more of the substance and contributes to the overall abuse. An obsession is a compulsive preoccupation with a fixed idea which may apply to the person who is dependent on chemical substances, but it is not a term used in this instance.

Questions

Psychiatry

A 33-year-old woman states that she finds it nearly impossible to visit friends, go to parties, or even to church. She has stood in front of a person's door and couldn't bring herself to knock because she feels inferior and thinks everyone is judging her. Even though she feels like she is productive on the job, she dreads talking to anyone in the department or attending department meetings because she knows they will ask her about her projects and the thought of speaking in front of co-workers makes her very anxious. This woman has a

(A) panic disorder
(B) personality disorder
(C) depression
(D) social phobia

Your Answer _____

_____

Correct Answers

A–307

(D) This is a classic description of someone with a social anxiety disorder or social phobia, the third largest mental health care problem in the world. Social phobia is the fear of social situations that involve interacting with other people. Cognitive-behavioral therapy is usually the best treatment.

Questions

Neurology/Infectious Disease

Mad cow disease is related to which similar degenerative brain disorder?

(A) Alzheimer's disease
(B) Creutzfeldt-Jakob disease
(C) Huntington's disease
(D) Parkinson's disease

Your Answer _____

Psychiatry/Neurology

The Mini-Mental State Examination (MMSE) is used to screen for

(A) cognitive impairment
(B) depression
(C) situational anxiety
(D) suicidal ideation

Your Answer _____

Correct Answers

A–308

(B) Mad cow disease (bovine spongiform encephalopathy) is an infectious disease in the brain of cattle. If humans eat diseased brain or spinal cord tissue from cattle, they may develop the human form of mad cow disease known as variant Creutzfeldt-Jakob disease.

A–309

(A) The MMSE is a 30-point questionnaire that is used to screen for cognitive impairment or dementia. It is also used to follow the course of cognitive changes over time.

Questions

Neurology/Anatomy

The part of the brain that controls voluntary movement and motor coordination, including posture is the

(A) pons
(B) cerebrum
(C) cerebellum
(D) brainstem

Your Answer _____

Emergency Medicine

Which of the following is more dangerous to the overall health of the patient?

(A) A greenstick fracture
(B) Torus fracture
(C) Pathologic fracture
(D) Sacroiliac joint fracture

Your Answer _____

Correct Answers

A–310

(C) The cerebellum helps coordinate balance and muscle coordination. Damage may result in ataxia.

A–311

(D) Sacroiliac (SI) joint fractures have the potential for serious consequences related to neurovascular injuries which may occur when the pelvis is rotated or crushed. A greenstick fracture is one seen in children and results from a bending force and involves only one cortex. A torus fracture, or buckle fracture, is very common in children. One side of the bone may buckle upon itself without disrupting the other side. A pathologic fracture occurs in a bone weakened by a pre-existing illness.

Questions

Emergency Medicine

Which of the following statements is/are true regarding compartment syndrome?

(A) It occurs most often in the forearm, hand, leg, and foot.
(B) It requires surgical consultation.
(C) Pain, paresthesias, and pallor are prominent signs/symptoms.
(D) All are true.

Your Answer _____

Psychiatry

While interviewing a patient, she becomes angry because you are wearing pearls like her mother used to wear. This patient is most probably displaying

(A) derealization
(B) depersonalization
(C) tangential thinking
(D) transference

Your Answer _____

Correct Answers

A–312

(D) All the statements are true regarding compartment syndrome, which occurs when pressure builds inside confined tissue, usually muscle, to dangerous levels.

A–313

(D) Transference refers to the unreasonable displacement of attitudes and feelings, which most commonly originate in childhood, to people in the here and now. Derealization refers to feelings that the external world seems different, unreal, or distant. Depersonalization is the sense that one is distanced from the environment or a spectator of one's own actions. Tangential thinking is an interruption in the patient's thought process followed by the patient talking about an apparently different topic.

Questions

Psychiatry

A lonely person develops a crush on another person, often a celebrity or prominent citizen, and often thinks that the object of the crush returns the same feelings. This abnormal thought process is described by the term

(A) somatic delusion
(B) delusion of nihilism
(C) erotic delusion
(D) delusion of grandeur

Your Answer _____

_____

Pulmonary

Pneumonia can be caused by a variety of bacterial and viral pathogens. Unique patient groups are susceptible to specific pathogens responsible for causing pneumonia. Of the pairs below, which is NOT responsible for pneumonia in the select population?

(A) Alcohol abuse   Klebsiella pneumonia
(B) Cystic fibrosis   Pseudomonas sp.
(C) Post-splenectomy   Meningococcal
(D) Children < 1 year old   RSV

Your Answer _____

_____

Correct Answers

A–314

(C) An erotic delusion arises out of fantasies. The person having an erotic delusion may bombard the object of his/her delusion with messages, phone calls, etc. A somatic delusion involves bizarre physical complaints possibly in an effort to explain somatic hallucinations. Delusion of nihilism causes the patient to have a hopeless outlook on life. Delusions of grandeur involve an inflated sense of self-importance.

A–315

(C) Pneumonia is an inflammation of the lung caused by viral, bacterial, and fungal microorganisms. There are certain subsets of the population with specific pneumonia causing pathogens based on their identifying features. Patients without a spleen are susceptible to encapsulated bacteria; however, meningococcal does not cause pneumonia.

Questions

Psychiatry

Which of the following is true regarding bipolar disorder?

(A) SSRIs are contraindicated in the treatment of mania.
(B) Bipolar II consists of alternating depressive symptoms and mania.
(C) Diagnosis is most common at age 30-40.
(D) Depression does not lead to suicidality in bipolar disorder.

Your Answer _____

_____

Gastrointestinal

A 19-year-old college student with a flu-like illness for two days presents to the student health clinic. You suspect influenza and examine her oropharynx, neck, chest, and abdomen. You palpate her liver edge about 2 cm below the costal margin. She is not jaundiced, has no history of liver disease and denies GI symptomatology. She had no evidence of splenomegaly. Your diagnosis now is

(A) influenza
(B) mononucleosis
(C) fatty liver secondary to alcohol intake
(D) mild hepatitis

Your Answer _____

_____

Correct Answers

A–316

(A) Bipolar disorder is a combination of mania, hypomania, and depression. Bipolar I includes mania alternating with depression. Bipolar II is hypomania alternating with depression and no episodes of mania are present. Bipolar disorder is often diagnosed for the first time in adolescence. Symptoms of mania include inflated self-esteem and grandiosity, decreased need for sleep, pressured speech, distractibility, excessive spending or other pleasurable activities with the potential for consequences. Depressive symptoms may include suicidal thoughts and acts. Treatment for depressive symptoms includes SSRI's; however, SSRIs are contraindicated in bipolar I as they can make mania worse.

A–317

(A) Identifying the liver edge in this young patient is likely a normal finding. If she had mononucleosis, she would more likely have an enlarged spleen which she does not. You could consider screening for excessive alcohol intake as she could have a fatty liver unrelated to the current illness. The most feasible diagnosis given the information already provided by the patient is still influenza.

Questions

Q–318

Neurology

A patient presents with apraxia, urinary incontinence, and dementia. This is a classic presentation of

(A) multifocal leukoencephalopathy
(B) Lewy-body dementia
(C) normal pressure hydrocephalus
(D) multi-infarct dementia

Your Answer _____

_____

Q–319

Women's Health

A 33-year-old woman presents with vaginal itching and discharge. Pelvic examination reveals a fishy malodorous, thin, gray vaginal discharge. The vaginal pH is 4.8. What would you expect to see on microscopic examination?

(A) Granulocytes and parabasal cells
(B) Yeast or hyphae
(C) Clue cells
(D) Motile, pear-shaped flagellated organisms

Your Answer _____

_____

Correct Answers

A–318

(C) Normal pressure hydrocephalus is due to altered spinal fluid dynamics that results in the symptoms presented. Multifocal leukoencephalopathy is seen in AIDS patients who have a progressive cognitive decline, motor dysfunction, and behavioral abnormalities. Lewy-body dementia presents with cognitive decline with confusion associated with hallucinations and mild motor abnormality. Multi-infarct dementia develops in a stepwise fashion and may not result in symptoms early; but, over time, as more areas of the brain are damaged, confusion, wandering, and problems with short-term memory occur.

A–319

(C) The findings are suggestive of bacterial vaginosis and clue cells would be present on microscopic examination. Granulocytes and parabasal cells occur in inflammatory vaginitis. Yeast or hyphae would be expected in a Candida infection and motile, pear-shaped flagellated organisms are present in trichamonal infection.

Questions

Psychiatry

After repeated exposure to many psychopharmacologic agents, individuals require a larger dose to produce intoxication of the magnitude that was experienced when the drug was first administered. This phenomenon is called

(A) addiction
(B) tachyphylaxis
(C) withdrawal
(D) tolerance

Your Answer _____

Neurology

Which of the following is indicative of an upper motor neuron lesion?

(A) Positive Babinski reflex
(B) Hyporeflexia
(C) Decreased muscle tone
(D) Fluctuating muscle weakness

Your Answer _____

Correct Answers

A–320

(D) This is the definition of tolerance. Addiction is a state in which the body relies on a substance for normal function and develops a physical or psychological dependence upon it. Tachyphylaxis is a term describing a rapid decrease in the response to a drug after repeated doses over a short period of time. Dependence occurs as a consequence of neuronal changes that develop after repeated exposure to an agent. Withdrawal describes a constellation of physiologic changes undergone by those who have become physically dependent of a chemical substance.

A–321

(A) A positive Babinski reflex is indicative of an upper motor neuron lesion. *Hyper*reflexia and *increased* motor tone would also be signs of upper motor neuron disease. Fluctuating muscle weakness relates to a neuromuscular junction disorder.

Questions

Psychiatry

Which one of the following is NOT a sign or symptom of *Cannabis* intoxication?

(A) Slowed reaction time
(B) Conjunctival injection
(C) Bradycardia
(D) Increased appetite

Your Answer _____

Gastrointestinal

Hiccups are repeated involuntary spasms of the diaphragm followed by sudden closure of the glottis, which checks the inflow of air and causes the characteristic sound. Transient hiccups are often caused by all of the following EXCEPT

(A) gastric distention
(B) alcohol consumption
(C) swallowing hot or irritating substances
(D) diaphragmatic pleurisy

Your Answer _____

Correct Answers

A–322

(C) With *Cannabis* intoxication, tachycardia is expected, not bradycardia.

A–323

(D) Diaphragmatic pleurisy is associated with intractable hiccups or hiccups that last more than one month.

Questions

Psychiatry

A 22-year-old patient brought to the emergency department is demonstrating psychomotor agitation, tremor, and vomiting. His blood pressure is elevated, and he is sweating. Shortly after arriving, he has a tonic-clonic seizure. This history is consistent with

(A) alcohol withdrawal
(B) acute myocardial infarction
(C) Tylenol overdose
(D) cocaine withdrawal

Your Answer _____

Psychiatry

The upper limit of urine detection for *Cannabis* is

(A) 12 hours
(B) 8 days
(C) 72 hours
(D) 4 weeks

Your Answer _____

Correct Answers

A–324

(A) Of the choices listed, alcohol withdrawal is the most likely diagnosis. Acute MI is unlikely as there is no history of chest pain and the patient is young for an MI. With Tylenol overdose, symptoms typically do not occur for about 24 hours post-ingestion. Cocaine withdrawal is marked by depression, fatigue, increased appetite, and craving.

A–325

(D) *Cannabis* can be detected in the urine for up to four weeks depending on how often the substance is used by the testee.

Questions

Pulmonary

You see a patient who complains of headache, sore throat, and postnasal drainage. On physical examination you describe cobble-stoning of the posterior oropharynx and pale, "boggy," swollen nasal mucosa. You diagnose allergic rhinitis. Which of the following medications is best at this point in time?

(A) Antibiotics, 10 day supply
(B) Antihistamine, second generation
(C) Decongestant
(D) NSAID

Your Answer _____

Radiology

You receive an X-ray report of a patient's hands and the report reads, "resorption of the tufts of the distal phalanges with malalignment and subluxation of joints known as opera glass hands." This is a typical report for the diagnosis of

(A) osteoarthritis
(B) rheumatoid arthritis
(C) psoriatic arthritis
(D) reactive arthritis

Your Answer _____

Correct Answers

A–326

(B) At this point in the patient's history, the best choice is an antihistamine. There is no evidence of infections, so antibiotics are not warranted. Similarly, NSAIDs might relieve the headache but will not address the allergies. Relieving the allergies should also relieve the headache.

A–327

(C) This is diagnostic for psoriatic arthritis.

Questions

Psychiatry

One recommended pharmacological treatment for a withdrawal syndrome from opioids includes

(A) diazepam
(B) phenobarbital
(C) clonidine
(D) bupropion

Your Answer _____

Emergency Medicine

How much time should elapse between a single scuba dive and air travel?

(A) 2 hours
(B) 12 hours
(C) 24 hours
(D) 36 hours

Your Answer _____

Correct Answers

A–328

(C) Clonidine is used in many treatment programs to lessen the severity of withdrawal symptoms from opioids. Diazepam or another benzodiazepine is used for alcohol withdrawal. Phenobarbital may be useful in those with CNS depression. Bupropion is helpful with nicotine withdrawal.

A–329

(B) Air travel after diving increases the risk of decompression sickness and air travel should not be undertaken for at least 12 hours after a single dive. After multiple dives or dives requiring decompression stops, air travel should not be undertaken for 24–48 hours.

Questions

Psychiatry

Which statement describes a somatic delusion?

(A) A belief that one's thoughts, feelings, or actions are being controlled by others.

(B) A belief that one is carrying a severe disease not supported by medical evidence.

(C) A belief that one's own thoughts can be read by others.

(D) A belief that the actions of others have a private meaning for the patient.

Your Answer _____

_____

Radiology/General Medicine

The association of the BRCA–1 gene (breast cancer gene) with other malignancies can be remembered by the mnemonic OCP (or COP). The C stands for

(A) colorectal cancer

(B) cerebellar cancer

(C) circulatory cancer (leukemias)

(D) chest cancer (various lung cancers)

Your Answer _____

_____

Correct Answers

A–330

(B) A somatic delusion is described by choice (B). Choice (A) describes a delusion of control; choice (C) describes thought broadcasting; and choice (D) a delusion of reference.

A–331

(A) The C stands for colorectal cancer. The O stands for ovarian and the P for prostate cancer.

Questions

Psychiatry

All of the following are signs of catatonia EXCEPT

(A) mutism
(B) rigidity
(C) staring
(D) lip smacking

Your Answer _____

_____

Psychiatry

Disorganized speech is believed to reflect an underlying impairment in thought process. Which description fits the classification of derailment speech?

(A) Speech that begins in a goal directed manner, but topics shift rapidly between sentences with no logical connection to the topic previously under discussion.
(B) Incomprehensible speech due to loss of logical connections between words, phrases, or sentences.
(C) Speech that begins in a goal directed manner, but deviates gradually and consistently such that answers to questions are not reached.
(D) Speech that is goal directed but excessive in unneeded detail. Direct answers are difficult to come by.

Your Answer _____

_____

Correct Answers

A–332

(D) While repetitive movements may be a sign of catatonia, lip smacking is typically not one of them.

A–333

(A) Derailment is described by choice (A). Choice (B) describes incoherence. Choice (C) describes tangentiality. Choice (D) describes circumstantiality.

Questions

Women's Health

A sexually active female presents with vulvar itching and burning, a copious vaginal discharge with a rancid odor, pain on urination and painful intercourse. Physical examination reveals a "frothy" thin, yellow-green discharge, and edema and erythema of the vulva. The diagnosis is

(A) *Candida* vaginitis
(B) Herpes vaginitis
(C) *Trichomonas* vaginitis
(D) gonorrhea

Your Answer _____

Psychiatry

A 37-year-old patient states that she has an ongoing love relationship with a famous Hollywood actor who doesn't live near the patient's home in eastern Pennsylvania. The patient is married and works as a secretary for the local water company. She seems to function normally in her everyday life. This patient most likely has

(A) schizophrenia
(B) delusional disorder
(C) schizoaffective disorder
(D) amnestic disorder

Your Answer _____

Correct Answers

A–334

(C) This is a typical presentation and findings for tricho-monal infection. A microscopic examination would reveal protozoa. *Candida* vaginitus presents with extreme itching and a cottage cheese-like discharge. Herpes vaginitis present with painful vesicular lesions. Gonorrhea presents with a greenish or yellow discharge from the cervix and is often asymptomatic in women.

A–335

(B) A delusional disorder has an onset between the age of 35–50 years in most cases. It is characterized by the persis-tence of delusions in the absence of hallucinations and dis-organized thoughts or behaviors. Patients do not typically experience significant changes in cognition. Schizophrenia is characterized by psychosis. The patient with a schizoaf-fective disorder exhibits symptoms consistent with schizo-phrenia but with superimposed episodes of depressive or manic symptoms. The patient with an amnestic disorder is unable to learn new information or recall previously learned facts or events.

Questions

Radiology/Musculoskeletal

A "night stick" fracture is a

(A) simple fracture through the middle of the ulna
(B) fracture of the distal humerus
(C) fracture of the radial head
(D) skull fracture

Your Answer _____

Psychiatry

Which statement is FALSE regarding cyclothymic disorders?

(A) They often begin in childhood or adolescence.
(B) There is a related family pattern of major depression and bipolar disorder.
(C) Alternating periods of hypomania with depression are characteristic.
(D) The predominant symptom seen in more than 75% of patients is hypomania.

Your Answer _____

Correct Answers

A–336

(A) A "night stick" fracture is a fracture of the ulna that gets its name from the injury that would occur if the patient were to have crossed his arms in front of his face for protection from the blow of a night stick and receive a fracture through the middle of the ulna. A fracture to the distal humerus or radial head often occurs from falling on an outstretched hand. A skull fracture may result from various types of trauma but this is not the definition of a "night stick" fracture.

A–337

(D) The predominant symptom in approximately 50% of patients is depression. A minority of patients have primarily hypomanic symptoms.

Questions

Psychiatry

Which disorder listed below is viewed by some as a disturbance of one of the phases of courtship? The disorder manifests as recurrent, intense sexually arousing fantasies, sexual images, or behaviors involving touching and rubbing against a nonconsenting person.

(A) Sexual fetishism
(B) Frotteurism
(C) Exhibitionism
(D) Sexual masochism

Your Answer _____

_____

Radiology/Emergency Medicine/ Musculoskeletal

The most common fracture of the forearm is a

(A) Colles' fracture
(B) boxer's fracture
(C) Bennett's fracture
(D) Rolando fracture

Your Answer _____

_____

Correct Answers

A–338

(B) Frotteurism is the term used to describe the disorder. Fetishism involves sexually arousing fantasies or behaviors involving the use of non-living objects or objects not associated with sexual arousal. Exhibitionism involves sexual arousal or fantasies involved with exposure of one's genitals to an unsuspecting stranger. Sexual masochism involves sexually arousing fantasies or behaviors involving the act of being humiliated, beaten, bound, or otherwise made to suffer.

A–339

(A) A Colles' fracture is a fracture of the distal radius received by falling on an outstretched hand. A Boxer's fracture is a fracture of the distal 5th metacarpal. A Bennett's fracture is a linear fracture at the base of the first metacarpal with intra-articular extension. A Rolando fracture is the same as a Bennett's fracture except the fracture is comminuted.

Questions

Psychiatry

A patient states that his left arm is paralyzed. When asked to move it, he states that he cannot. He appears depressed about this problem. On physical examination you demonstrate the presence of deep tendon reflexes, and nerve conduction studies are normal. You suspect a diagnosis of

(A) a conversion disorder
(B) malingering
(C) hypochondriasis
(D) Either (A) or (B)

Your Answer _____

EENT

The "thumb" sign seen on a lateral X-ray view of the neck indicates a diagnosis of

(A) discitis at C3-C4
(B) epiglottitis
(C) croup
(D) retropharyngeal abscess

Your Answer _____

Correct Answers

A–340

(A) A conversion disorder symptom mimics dysfunction in the voluntary motor or sensory system; but with clinical evaluation, the symptoms prove to be nonphysiologic. Malingering is a deliberate production of disease or exaggeration of symptoms for secondary gain. Hypochondriasis is a preoccupation with fears of having a serious disease based on the patient's misinterpretation of bodily symptoms.

A–341

(B) The presence of a "thumb" sign is indicative of epiglottitis. An X-ray of discitis would show inflammation in the disc space of the involved vertabrae indicating infection. With croup, an X-ray of neck soft tissue reveals subglottic narrowing. X-ray findings for retropharyngeal abscess are not very specific.

Questions

Musculoskeletal

Which of the following is NOT a clinical feature of compartment syndrome?

(A) Pulselessness, pallor, paresthesia, pain, and poikilothermia

(B) Normal compartment pressures are <10 mmHg.

(C) Nerve dysfunction is followed by pain.

(D) Delta pressure of > 10-35 mmHg are abnormal.

Your Answer _____

_____

Emergency Medicine

What chest X-ray findings would you expect to see in a patient with a tension pneumothorax?

(A) A very thin white line with no lung markings beyond that line

(B) A contralateral mediastinal shift

(C) A dark and expanded hemithorax of the involved lung

(D) All of the above would be seen.

Your Answer _____

_____

Correct Answers

A-342

(C) Compartment syndrome occurs when there is increased pressure in a limited space such as the forearm or lower leg. The increased pressure compresses blood flow and nerve resulting in the 5 P's: pulselessness, pallor, paresthesia, pain and poikilothermia. Pain is the first symptom, followed later by nerve dysfunction. Diagnosis is made by measuring the pressure in the affected area using a handheld manometer or by measuring the delta pressure; the difference between diastolic blood pressure and the pressure of the tissue in the compartment.

A-343

(D) All of the findings listed would be present in a tension pneumothorax.

Questions

Emergency Medicine

The correct position for an endotracheal tube is that the tip should be

(A) in the right mainstem bronchus
(B) in the left mainstem bronchus
(C) 2–6 cm above the carina
(D) 2–6 cm below the carina

Your Answer _____

Emergency Medicine

Indications for ordering plain abdominal X-rays include which of the following?

(A) Bowel obstruction
(B) Viscus perforation
(C) Foreign body ingestion
(D) All of the above

Your Answer _____

Correct Answers

A–344

(C) A correctly placed endotracheal tube will be 2–6 cm above the carina.

A–345

(D) Plain abdominal films would be the first study to order. CT will likely be needed if an organ is perforated to determine management.

Questions

Cardiovascular

All of the following are causes of lymphedema EXCEPT

(A) traumatic
(B) infective
(C) inflammatory
(D) neurogenic

Your Answer _____

Gastrointestinal

A 67-year-old female presents to the ED with abdominal pain. She rates the pain as a 10/10 and it started suddenly 2 hours ago. She denies nausea, vomiting, fevers, diarrhea, or constipation. PMH is significant for CAD with MI 2 years ago. Abdominal exam is mildly tender but out of proportion to the amount of pain she is experiencing. What imaging test would confirm the diagnosis?

(A) Flat and upright abdominal X-ray
(B) CT with IV and oral contrast
(C) CT Angiography
(D) Surgical exploration

Your Answer _____

Correct Answers

A-346

(D) The answer that is not a cause of lymphedema is neurogenic. Causes of lymphedema can be remembered by the mnemonic CTIN, where C = congenital; T = traumatic; I = Infective/Inflammatory; and N = neoplastic.

A-347

(C) The most likely diagnosis is acute mesenteric ischemia (AMI). AMI presents with sudden onset of severe abdominal pain out of proportion to exam findings, and AMI is most common in those with cardiovascular disease. Chronic mesenteric ischemia presents as abdominal angina, with pain occurring 10 to 30 minutes after eating. Abdominal X-ray and CT will rule out other causes of abdominal pain, and CT with oral contrast may obscure the mesenteric vessels. Angiography will outline the vasculature of the abdomen and mesentary. While surgery may be indicated for treatment, it is not an imaging test.

Questions

Cardiovascular/Pharmacology

Which statement is NOT true about the use of clonidine in the treatment of hypertension?

(A) It reduces central sympathetic outflow.
(B) It is associated with elevation in LDL cholesterol.
(C) Dry mouth and sedation are common side effects.
(D) It can be used with vasodilators.

Your Answer _____

Urology/Renal

A 42-year-old male presents to the clinic with bilateral flank pain for 2 months. It is constant and there are no precipitating or alleviating factors. Urinalysis reveals 2+ blood, CBC reveals a slight anemia, and ultrasound shows bilateral, thin-walled, fluid-filled cysts. Based on this information, which of the following is true?

(A) You would expect the creatinine and blood pressure to be normal
(B) Ultrasound findings also include cysts on the liver and pancreas.
(C) Use of ace-inhibitor medications will successfully treat this patient's underlying condition.
(D) Transplanted kidneys will also develop cysts.

Your Answer _____

Correct Answers

A–348

(B) Clonidine is not associated with elevations in LDL cholesterol. Thiazide diuretics, which are often used together with clonidine, do cause elevations in lipids. The other statements are true.

A–349

(B) Polycystic kidney disease (PKD) is characterized by the growth of thin-walled, fluid-filled cysts in the kidneys. PKD is associated with hematuria, hypertension, and recurrent urinary tract infections. The most common symptom is back and flank pain due in part to the enlarged kidney. There is no cure, and treatment is supportive. Hypertension is controlled with the use of ACE-I or ARB. Transplantation may be considered in those with renal failure, and transplanted kidneys do not develop cysts. There are extra-renal manifestations of PKD such as cysts in the liver and pancreas.

Questions

Gastrointestinal/Oncology

Patients with gastric cancer will likely have which blood group?

(A) A
(B) B
(C) AB
(D) O

Your Answer _____

_____

Radiology

In reading a chest X-ray, you note "superior surface notch of the ribs." This raises suspicion of all of the following EXCEPT

(A) coarctation of the aorta
(B) hyperparathyroidism
(C) neurofibromatosis
(D) a connective tissue disorder

Your Answer _____

_____

Correct Answers

A–350

(A) Patients will likely have blood group A. In fact, to remember the characteristics of gastric cancer, one can remember the 4 A's: Anorexia, Anemia, Asthenia, Blood Group A.

A–351

(A) Coarctation of the aorta is suspected when one sees an "inferior surface notch of the ribs."

Questions

Q-352

Cardiovascular

You see a patient in the emergency department who is complaining of an abrupt onset of chest pain. He describes the pain as a heavy sensation behind and to the left of the sternum. There is no radiation of the pain, he has no associated diaphoresis. He prefers to be sitting on the exam table leaning forward slightly and the pain significantly worsens if he is lying flat. What EKG findings do you expect to see in this patient?

(A) ST elevation in most leads
(B) ST depression in most leads
(C) A shortened PR interval
(D) An elongated QT interval

Your Answer _____

Q-353

Pediatrics

One of the following statements is INCORRECT regarding mothers who are breastfeeding their babies. Which one?

(A) It is acceptable for the mother to eat spicy foods while breastfeeding.
(B) Lactation amenorrhea prevents a pregnancy during the time of breastfeeding.
(C) Smoking will increase the number of respiratory infections in the nursing baby.
(D) Alcohol, no more than 2 ounces/day, is safe during breastfeeding.

Your Answer _____

Correct Answers

A–352

(A) This clinical scenario describes pericarditis. The classic EKG finding in pericarditis is diffuse ST elevation in many leads, not following any particular pattern. A shortened PR interval is associated with Wolf Parkinson White, which leads to tachyarrhythmias. An elongated QT interval is also associated with tachyarrhythmias.

A–353

(B) Most breastfeeding women have abnormal menstrual periods. This phenomenon is called lactation amenorrhea, and although the risk of pregnancy is less during this time, it still can occur.

Questions

General Medicine/Pharmacology

A 70-year-old man presents with bleeding from the gums. He had a coronary artery bypass graft at age 67. His only medication is aspirin which he has taken for three years with no problems. A drug history reveals that he began taking an over-the-counter herbal supplement six weeks prior to this bleeding episode. You suspect a drug interaction as the explanation for his problem. Which OTC herbal remedy is known to cause spontaneous bleeding, as well as interactions with anticoagulant and antiplatelet drugs.

(A) St. John's wort
(B) Ginkgo biloba
(C) Kava
(D) Ma huang

Your Answer _____

_____

Correct Answers

(B)   Ginkgo biloba is promoted to improve cognitive functioning and increase blood flow. It may also cause bleeding and interact with anticoagulant and antiplatelet drugs.

Questions

Musculoskeletal

Spondyloarthritis shows major differences among various ethnic groups, with Japanese and African populations rarely being affected. Laboratory evidence strongly suggests the participation of which gene in the pathogenesis of this disorder?

(A) HLA–B27
(B) HLA–B13
(C) HLA–C6
(D) HLA–B38

Your Answer _____

_____

Correct Answers

(A) The HLA–B27 allele is strongly suggestive of pathogenesis of this disorder and other arthritic disorders. The other three genes listed may predispose a person to psoriasis and psoriatic arthritis.

Questions

Musculoskeletal

A patient presents with a history of low back pain for more than three months duration. The pain is alleviated by exercise and is not relieved by rest. He also complains of restricted lumbar spinal motion. During the physical examination, the patient is noted to have decreased chest expansion relative to normal values for age and sex. A radiograph of the spine reveals sacroiliitis. This constellation of findings meets the criteria for a diagnosis of

(A) rheumatoid arthritis of the spine
(B) Osteoarthritis of the spine
(C) ankylosing spondylitis
(D) systemic lupus erythematosis

Your Answer _____

Musculoskeletal/Rheumatology

This disorder is a chronic autoimmune illness characterized by autoantibodies directed at nuclear antigens and causing a variety of symptoms, including rash, arthritis, fever, nephritis, and neurologic disease. It is

(A) rheumatoid arthritis
(B) systemic lupus erythematosis
(C) Polyarteritis nodosa
(D) Wegener granulomatosis

Your Answer _____

Correct Answers

A–356

(C) The description meets the New York criteria for ankylosing spondylitis. Rheumatoid arthritis more commonly affects the cervical spine and spares the lumbar and sacral spine. Osteoarthritis of the spine causes cartilage to be worn between subsequent vertebrae which rub together, causing pain, swelling, and loss of motion of the joint. Systemic lupus erythematosis produces various joint symptoms, ranging from intermittent arthralgias to acute polyarthritis, but it typically does not cause major spinal problems.

A–357

(B) The correct answer is systemic lupus erythematosis. The genetic makeup of an individual plays a major role in susceptibility to rheumatoid arthritis. No single etiologic factor accounts for all causes of R.A. In polyarteritis nodosa, one sees a necrotizing medium-sized vessel arteritis. Wegener's granulomatosis is relatively uncommon. It is characterized by necrotizing granulomatous inflammation and vasculitis of small- and medium-sized blood vessels.

Questions

Rheumatology

Scleroderma is a slowly progressive rheumatic disease characterized by deposition of fibrous connective tissue in the skin and other tissues. Which of the following may be components of scleroderma?

(A) Raynaud's phenomenon
(B) Distal interphalangeal bone destruction
(C) Esophageal hypomotility
(D) All of the above are characteristics of scleroderma.

Your Answer _____

_____

Musculoskeletal/Rheumatology

Idiopathic inflammatory myopathies primarily affect skeletal muscle. A patient showing symmetrical proximal muscle weakness in all extremities accompanied by a deep red skin rash on the extensor surfaces of the hands and knees is likely suffering from

(A) dermatomyositis
(B) polymyositis
(C) rhabdomyolysis
(D) polymyalgia rheumatica

Your Answer _____

_____

Correct Answers

A–358

(D) All may be components of scleroderma, as well as swelling and thickening of the fingers and hands.

A–359

(A) Dermatomyositis is a connective tissue disease characterized by inflammation of the muscles and skin. Polymyositis is an idiopathic inflammatory myopathy that causes symmetric proximal muscle weakness but does not have the rash. Rhabdomyolysis is a breakdown of muscle cells, which may be from various causes. Polymyalgia rheumatica is a disease of the elderly and often seen in patients with underlying osteoarthritis. Pain is typically localized to the shoulder and hip girdles.

Questions

Rheumatology

A small vessel vasculitis more common in children than adults and manifested by purpura, urticaria, abdominal pain, gastrointestinal bleeding, intussusception, arthralgias, and glomerulonephritis is likely

(A) Churg-Strauss syndrome
(B) Wegener's granulomatosis
(C) Henoch-Schönlein purpura
(D) urticarial vasculitis

Your Answer _____

Rheumatology

A 53-year-old patient presents with proximal muscle pain worse at night and in the early morning. She also complains of fever, recent onset headache, and masticatory muscle claudication. Lab studies indicate an elevation of acute phase reactants. Among the disorders listed, which is the top suspicion?

(A) Polyarteritis nodosa
(B) Microscopic polyangiitis
(C) Giant cell arteritis
(D) Atherosclerosis obliterans

Your Answer _____

Correct Answers

A–360

(C) Henoch-Schönlein purpura presents as a classic triad of purpura, arthritis, and abdominal pain. It is usually self-limiting but may progress to irreversible kidney damage. Churg-Strauss syndrome is an allergic granulomatosis angiitis which affects small and medium arteries and veins and is also associated with bronchial asthma. Wegener's granulomatosis is characterized by necrotizing granulomatous inflammation of small- and medium-sized vessels. Urticarial vasculitis presents as wheals or serpentine papules.

A–361

(C) The presentation of the patient, both age and symptoms, is suggestive of giant cell arteritis. It almost always occurs in people over the age of 50 and causes the symptoms as well as visual disturbances in some. The new onset headache and jaw claudication may allow for a presumptive diagnosis in the absence of biopsy. Polyarteritis nodosa also occurs in the 4th and 5th decades and is more common in men than women. Patients present with fever, sweats, weight loss, and severe muscle and joint aches/pains. Microscopic polyangiitis affects individuals of any age group and can affect many of the body's organ systems, including the kidneys, nervous system, skin, and lungs. Atherosclerosis obliterans refers to narrowing and gradual blockage of arteries. The symptoms will depend on the location of the arteries affected and how severe the blockage is but usually consist of muscle pain, cold extremities, and if arteries in the legs are involved, numbness, weakness, and walking problems.

Questions

EENT/Mouth

A 66-year-old female presents with a history of an increasing burning sensation of the tongue when she eats sharp-tasting foods. She also states that her tongue has become red and shiny. She wears both upper and lower dentures. You diagnose atrophic glossitis and suspect the cause to be

(A) nutritional
(B) infectious
(C) mechanical
(D) neurological

Your Answer _____

Endocrinology/Dermatology

A 14-year-old female presents to the clinic complaining of darkening skin around her neck, on her elbows, and in her armpits. The skin also appears thickened. Physical examination reveals the patient to be hypertensive and overweight. Her family history is positive for diabetes mellitus. The diagnosis is

(A) hypomelanosis
(B) acanthosis nigricans
(C) melasma
(D) diabetic dermopathy

Your Answer _____

Correct Answers

A–362

(A) The most likely cause is a lack of B vitamins in the diet. A daily supplement with folic acid, niacin, B-12, pyridoxine, and riboflavin may relieve the symptoms. In a person of this age, a daily multi-vitamin, multi-mineral supplement would be advisable. An infectious etiology could be the presence of yeast, which is not uncommon in older persons with weakened immune systems. What makes this unlikely is that there is no evidence of a white coating on the tongue which can be scraped off. A third, more remote possibility in this particular patient, is a mechanical injury secondary to abrasion of the tongue as it contacts the dentures. The history is not consistent with this diagnosis. One would need more history to indicate a neurological problem. This is the least likely answer.

A–363

(B) Acanthosis nigricans is a skin disease characterized by hyperpigmentation and hyperkeratosis particularly of the skin folds. It is associated with insulin resistance and prediabetes and responds to weight loss and life style changes, particularly healthy food choices. Hypomelanosis refers to a lack of skin color, which is opposite to what the patient describes. Melasma, common during pregnancy, is an acquired hypermelanosis of sun-exposed areas. The cheeks, upper lip, chin and forehead are the most common locations. Diabetic dermopathy is a skin condition characteristic of diabetes and it presents as light brown or reddish oval or round scaly patches, most often on the shins or front of the thighs and less often on the scalp and trunk.

Questions

Renal-Urology/Geriatrics/Pharmacology

A 72-year-old man with hypertension complains of urinary hesitancy, nocturia, frequency and decreased force and caliber of his urinary stream. He is presumed to have benign prostatic hypertrophy (BPH). Which drug would treat both the hypertension and the BPH?

(A) Lisinopril
(B) Diltiazem
(C) Prazosin
(D) Hydralazine

Your Answer _____

Women's Health/Pharmacology

A 20-year-old woman presents with a malodorous vaginal discharge. A saline wet prep reveals WBCs, bacteria, and clue cells. A KOH prep gives a positive "whiff" test. The best treatment for this disorder is

(A) fluconazole
(B) metronidazole
(C) famciclovir
(D) doxycycline

Your Answer _____

Correct Answers

A–364

(C) Prazosin is an alpha-adrenergic antagonist and would treat both conditions. None of the other drugs would do the same.

A–365

(B) The patient has bacterial vaginosis for which metronidazole is the drug of choice. Fluconazole is used to treat vaginitis secondary to yeast infections. Famciclovir is an antiviral agent used to treat herpes genitalis, and doxycycline is useful in infections caused by chlamydia.

Questions

Women's Health/OB-GYN

An Rh-negative mother is pregnant with her first baby. You have put a note in her chart to alert everyone involved with the patient that the mother should receive Rh immune globulin (Rho-Gam) after delivery. Within what time frame should the Rho-Gam be administered?

(A) 12 hours
(B) 36 hours
(C) 72 hours
(D) one week

Your Answer _____

Emergency Medicine

Traumatic injury to the deep peroneal nerve could result in a(n)

(A) inability to evert the foot
(B) inability to extend the knee
(C) inability to dorsiflex the foot
(D) loss of sensation to the sole of the foot

Your Answer _____

Correct Answers

A–366

(C) Rho-Gam is most effective if administered within 72 hours after delivery. The mother should also receive a dose at approximately 28 weeks of the pregnancy.

A–367

(C) The deep peroneal nerve descends to the front of the ankle joint, where it divides into a lateral and a medial terminal branch. Trauma to the nerve can result in an inability to dorsiflex the foot. Damage to the superficial peroneal nerve could result in an inability to evert the foot. The femoral nerve is associated with extension of the knee. Loss of sensation to the sole of the foot implies tibial nerve dysfunction.

Questions

Emergency Medicine

Movement of fracture pieces perpendicular to the long axis of bone is descriptive of which kind of fracture?

(A) Angulation
(B) Spiral
(C) Displacement
(D) Stress

Your Answer _____

Hematology/Pharmacology

Pick the true statement below.

(A) Warfarin has a quick onset of action; once administration is stopped, the prothrombin time returns to normal within 48 hours.
(B) A pregnant woman who gets a DVT should be quickly anticoagulated using heparin and then maintained on warfarin for the duration of her pregnancy.
(C) A patient taking cholestyramine cannot take warfarin concomitantly.
(D) Amiodarone inhibits the metabolism of warfarin.

Your Answer _____

Correct Answers

A–368

(C) A displacement fracture is one in which the two ends of the broken bone are separated from one another. An angulated fracture is one in which the fragments of bone are at angles to one another. A spiral fracture, also called a torsion fracture, is one in which the bone has been twisted apart. A stress fracture is caused by repeated application of a heavy load, such as seen in gymnasts, runners, and dancers.

A–369

(D) Amiodarone inhibits the metabolism of warfarin by interfering with the cytochrome P450 enzyme system. Warfarin has a slow onset of action—taking about five days to become fully effective. Warfarin is also teratogenic and should not be used in pregnant women. Cholestyramine interferes with intestinal absorption of warfarin and if given to the same patient, administration must be after two hours or more.

Questions

Pulmonary/Pharmacology

A patient presents with pain in the right shoulder for two days duration. During the history you learn that the pain is localized, sharp, and fleeting and is made worse by coughing, sneezing, and moving. This pain will be treated with

(A) a codeine-containing cough syrup
(B) an NSAID
(C) acetaminophen plus a sling
(D) antibiotics and acetaminophen

Your Answer _____

Emergency Medicine

Firemen rescued a woman from a burning building. Her entire chest, head, and neck were severely burned. The estimated body surface area of burns is

(A) 27%
(B) 9%
(C) 18%
(D) 13%

Your Answer _____

Correct Answers

A–370

(B) The pain the patient is experiencing describes pleurisy. Pleuritic pain will respond best to an NSAID. A cough syrup containing codeine may lessen the cough and indirectly help the pain, but it won't directly help the pleurisy. Putting the arm in a sling won't be helpful as the pain is referred from involvement of the diaphragm. Pleurisy is not an infective process; therefore, antibiotics are not indicated.

A–371

(C) One uses the rule of 9's when estimating percentage of body burn. The entire chest is 9% and the entire head and neck is 9%. Therefore, the correct answer is (C), 18%.

Questions

Endocrinology

A 32-year-old female presents to the clinic with concerns of central obesity, amenorrhea, and kidney stones. On physical exam you note a round face and an accumulation of fat on the upper back and lower neck. She has central obesity and stick-like extremities. Based on the most likely diagnosis, all of the following are true EXCEPT

(A) Overnight dexamethasone suppression test will result in an elevated plasma cortisol.
(B) May be caused from a pituitary tumor, adrenal tumor, small cell lung cancer, or excess oral glucocorticoids.
(C) Specific signs are proximal muscle weakness and pigmented striae greater than 1 cm wide.
(D) Need to watch for a crisis: hypotension, vomiting, diarrhea, dehydration, and mental status changes.

Your Answer _____

Cardiovascular

In examining the heart of a 39-year-old woman who complains of chest pain, you hear a mid-systolic click. You will refer her for echocardiography, but suspect the diagnosis will be

(A) mitral valve prolapse
(B) mitral regurgitation
(C) aortic stenosis
(D) pericarditis

Your Answer _____

Correct Answers

A–372

(D) Cushing's disease is caused by an excess of gluco-corticoids, commonly from mediations, but also from an excess of ACTH from the pituitary, adrenal gland, or non-pituitary ACTH secreting tumors such as small cell lung cancer. Common PE findings include moon facies, buffalo hump, supraclavicular fat pads, darkened striae, and proximal muscle weakness. Lab testing reveals an elevated 24-hour urinary cortisol and an elevated cortisol following an overnight dexamethasone suppression test. A gluco-corticoid insufficiency, Addison's disease, may result in an adrenal crisis that may be life-threatening if not treated.

A–373

(A) A mid-systolic click is the hallmark of mitral valve prolapse. The classic murmur of mitral regurgitation is a high-pitched holosystolic murmur. Aortic stenosis produces a mid-systolic ejection murmur heard best in the aortic area. Pericarditis is an inflammation of the pericardium and may produce a friction rub.

Questions

Q–374

Hematology

A 19-year-old female patient presents with fatigue, tachypnea on exertion, palpitations, brittle nails, and cheilosis. When questioned, she admits to mild dysphagia and a craving for ice. From this history, you suspect

(A) a thyroid disorder
(B) an eating disorder
(C) a vitamin deficiency
(D) anemia

Your Answer _____

Q–375

Gastrointestinal/Pharmacology

What is the role of HMG-CoA reductase inhibitors on hyperlipidemia?

(A) They cause catabolism of VLDLs and chylomicrons.
(B) They bind negatively charged bile acids.
(C) They decrease cholesterol absorption and thus increase the hepatocyte surface-LDL receptors
(D) They do none of the above.

Your Answer _____

Correct Answers

A–374

(D) This is a classic presentation for someone with iron deficiency anemia who exhibits pica, or a craving for non-nutritive substances—in this case, ice. Hypothyroid may cause fatigue, but the other symptoms do not support it. There is no evidence of an eating disorder. Certain vitamin deficiencies can cause cheilosis, but the rest of the history doesn't support this diagnosis.

A–375

(D) Reductase inhibitors interfere with cholesterol formation and thereby decrease total cholesterol, LDL-cholesterol, VLDL, and triglycerides. Niacin causes catabolism of VLDLs and chylomicrons. Bile-acid binding resins, like cholestyramine, bind bile acids and lead to enhanced conversion of cholesterol to bile acids and ultimately lower the cholesterol level. Ezetimibe is an example of a drug that inhibits intestinal absorption of cholesterol.

Questions

Cardiology/Emergency Medicine

A patient is in ventricular fibrillation. The initial setting for a monophasic defibrillator is 200 joules. If the patient does NOT respond, what is the next recommended setting?

(A) 100 joules
(B) 200 joules
(C) 200–300 joules
(D) 360 joules

Your Answer _____

Hematology

A 45-year-old male presents with fatigue, night sweats, and a low-grade fever. On physical examination, he has an enlarged spleen. His laboratory studies returns a white blood count of 150,000/mL, with normal red cell and platelet morphology. The vitamin B12 level and uric acid are slightly elevated. A *bcr-abl* gene was found in peripheral blood. The diagnosis is

(A) acute myelogenous leukemia
(B) chronic myelogenous leukemia
(C) chronic lymphocytic leukemia
(D) acute lymphoblastic leukemia

Your Answer _____

Correct Answers

A–376

(C) Monophasic machine settings typically are 50, 100, 200, and 300 joules. If starting with 200 joules and there is no response, some say that you can shock again with 200 J and then the next setting should be 300 joules.

A–377

(B) The description is typical for chronic myelogenous leukemia, which occurs in middle age and is noted for having the Philadelphia chromosome or *bcr-abl* gene. Acute myelogenous leukemia is the most common type of acute leukemia. It is characterized by the production of *blast* cells. Chronic lymphocytic leukemia is a malignancy of B lymphocytes and manifests clinically by immunosuppression, bone marrow failure, and organ infiltration with lymphocytes. Acute lymphoblastic leukemia is characterized by immature white blood cells that are overproduced in the bone marrow.

Questions

Endocrine/Oncology

The most common tumor of the pituitary is a

(A) prolactinoma
(B) pituitary adenoma
(C) ACTH-producing tumor
(D) non-functioning tumor

Your Answer _____

_____

Cardiology

Which one of the following is a sign of left ventricular failure?

(A) JVD
(B) Hepatomegaly
(C) Ascites
(D) Gallop rhythm

Your Answer _____

_____

Correct Answers

A–378

(A) Prolactinoma account for approximately 30% of all pituitary tumors. In general, pituitary tumors are classified according to their production of specific hormones with one exception: the non-functioning tumor which is a hormonally inactive adenoma.

A–379

(D) Persons in left ventricular failure may develop a gallop rhythm which is indicative of increased intracardiac pressure. JVD, hepatomegaly, and ascites are signs of right-sided heart failure.

Questions

Cardiology/Anatomy

A patient has suffered a posterior wall myocardial infarction. Which artery is most commonly occluded?

(A) Right coronary artery
(B) Left circumflex coronary artery
(C) Left main coronary artery
(D) Posterior coronary artery

Your Answer _____

Musculoskeletal

A patient reports severe pain on the bottom of her left foot in the morning which mostly subsides after a few minutes of walking. Palpation over the heel produces pain. An X-ray was noncontributory. Her diagnosis is

(A) an anterior talofibular ligament sprain
(B) plantar fasciitis
(C) tarsal tunnel syndrome
(D) fat pad syndrome

Your Answer _____

Correct Answers

A–380

(B) Most posterior wall MIs are due to occlusion of the left circumflex coronary artery, although a small percentage can be caused by a blocked right coronary artery. Total occlusion of the left main coronary artery is associated with a high degree of fatality from an anterior MI. Only 4% of people have a posterior coronary artery, which diminishes its overall frequency of participation in myocardial infarction rates.

A–381

(B) This is a typical presentation for plantar fasciitis, an inflammatory disorder of the fascia in the foot. Tarsal tunnel syndrome presents with more diffuse symptoms over the plantar surface. A patient with a fat pad syndrome will have pain concentrated over the center of the heel that feels like a deep bruise. A patient with an anterior talofibular ligament sprain should give a history of a recent injury.

Questions

Cardiovascular

A patient complains of aching pain in the lower right leg when walking, which is consistent with a history of intermittent claudication. Which imaging technique is most used in the diagnosis of this arterial disorder?

(A) Doppler ultrasound
(B) Magnetic resonance angiography
(C) Ankle-brachial index
(D) Computed tomography angiography

Your Answer _____

_____

Renal/Urinary/Pharmacology

A 73-year-old woman presents with a history of classic urge incontinence. Appropriate treatment is

(A) topical estrogen cream
(B) culpo-cystourethropexy
(C) alpha adrenergic antagonist
(D) anticholinergic agent

Your Answer _____

_____

Correct Answers

A–382

(C) A Doppler ultrasound is used to image the venous system. A calculation called the ankle-brachial index is used to diagnose peripheral arterial disease in patients with and without symptoms. Magnetic resonance angiography is an alternative to the Doppler study but usually involves the injection of a dye to get a better study. Computed tomography angiography uses X-rays to visualize blood flow and is very reliable.

A–383

(D) Urge incontinence is treated medically rather than surgically. Anticholinergic (antispasmodic) drugs are effective. Stress incontinence may be associated with hypoestrogenism of the vagina or urethra, and in such cases, topical estrogen creams are indicated. If the bladder neck has descended below the midportion of the pubic symphysis, a culpo-cystourethropexy can pull the bladder neck into proper position. Alpha adrenergic antagonists are useful in treating benign prostatic hypertrophy.

Questions

Psychiatry

Sexual sadism is the attainment of sexual arousal by inflicting pain upon the sexual object. Sadism belongs to which of the following psychosexual disorders?

(A) Gender identity disorder
(B) Psychosexual dysfunction
(C) Paraphilias
(D) Disorders of sexual desire

Your Answer _____

_____

Psychiatry

A patient presents to your practice in psychiatry. He appears selfish, callous, and impulsive and admits to having had repeated legal problems. He also admits to promiscuity. Based only on these criteria, he is best classified as having which type of personality disorder?

(A) Narcissistic
(B) Antisocial
(C) Passive-aggressive
(D) Schizoid

Your Answer _____

_____

Correct Answers

A–384

(C) Sadism belong to the psychosexual disorders known as paraphilias or sexual arousal disorders in which the excitement stage of sexual activity is associated with sexual objects or orientations different from those usually associated with adult heterosexual stimulation. Gender identity disorders include transsexualism and homosexuality. Psychosexual dysfunctions include problems such as impotence, vaginismus, frigidity, etc. Disorders of sexual desire consist of diminished or absent libido in either sex and may be a function of organic or psychologic difficulties.

A–385

(B) The criteria fit the antisocial personality type. Failure to learn from experiences is evident in his repeated legal problems. The narcissistic personality type may be an exhibitionist, have grandiose ideas, and be preoccupied with power while lacking interest in others. The passive-aggressive individual is often stubborn, procrastinating, argumentative, clinging, and negative to authority figures. The schizoid personality is shy, introverted, and withdrawn and avoids close relationships.

Questions

Psychiatry/Pharmacology

Your patient with bipolar disorder has been well controlled with lithium carbonate for several years. She recently returned from an extended stay in Florida. While in Florida, she was noted to have hypertension and has been taking HCTZ for the past month. Today, she complains of nervousness, tremor, muscle weakness, vomiting, and confusion. The most helpful laboratory study is a(n)

(A) CBC
(B) electrolyte panel
(C) serum lithium level
(D) potassium level

Your Answer _____

_____

Correct Answers

A–386

(C) This patient has evidence of toxic levels of lithium brought on by the administration of HCTZ, which causes potassium loss. While a potassium level would also be important, it is not the most beneficial laboratory study. There is no indication for ordering a CBC.

Questions

Hematology

A 60-year-old woman presents with back pain of several months duration but also with an acute pain in her right hip. She appears pale and has tenderness upon palpation of the thoracic spine and with movement of the right leg. Laboratory studies reveal hypercalcemia, elevated sedimentation rate, and anemia. Radiologic studies confirm a fracture of the femoral neck and multiple compression fractures of the spine. Her bone marrow was infiltrated by plasma cells. A serum protein electrophoresis showed the presence of paraproteins with a monoclonal spike visible in the gamma globulin region. The most likely diagnosis is

(A) multiple myeloma
(B) monoclonal gammopathy of unknown significance (MGUS)
(C) Waldenström's macroglobulinemia
(D) amyloidosis

Your Answer _____

Correct Answers

A–387

(A) The most likely diagnosis is multiple myeloma, which often presents with back pain or a pathologic fracture. Anemia is a common finding. It is one of a group of disorders known as plasma cell neoplasms. The presence of plasma cells in the bone marrow are a helpful finding, but the hallmark of myeloma is the finding of paraprotein on serum protein electrophoresis. Monoclonal gammopathy is more common than multiple myeloma. Persons having this diagnosis have the presence of a monoclonal immunoglobulin in the serum or urine but have no evidence of multiple myeloma. Waldenström's macroglobulinemia is a rare type of plasma cell neoplasm. The abnormal plasma cells invade the bone marrow, lymph nodes, and spleen and produce excessive amounts of IgM which causes hyperviscosity of the blood. Amyloidosis refers to a variety of conditions in which amyloid proteins are abnormally deposited in tissues or organs.

Questions

Q–388

Cardiovascular

The most common sustained cardiac dysrhythmia affecting more than 2 million people in the United States is

(A) Mobitz type I block
(B) PSVT
(C) atrial fibrillation
(D) premature ventricular contractions (PVCs)

Your Answer _____

_____

Q–389

Cardiovascular/Pharmacology

Patients with cardiac dysrhythmias can have rhythm restored with medication, electrical shocks, or a combination of both. Some medications can be used for cardioversion and others for maintenance of sinus rhythm. All of the following drugs can be used for cardioversion of atrial fibrillation or flutter. Of the drugs listed, which one is contraindicated in a patient with atrial dysrhythmia and concomitant heart failure?

(A) Amiodarone
(B) Dofetilide
(C) Digoxin
(D) Propafenone

Your Answer _____

_____

Correct Answers

A–388

(C) Atrial fibrillation is the most common sustained dysrhythmia with nearly 2 million people in the United States being affected by it. Nearly 3% of patients with underlying heart disease develop some form of AV block. A Mobitz type I AV block is often nonprogressive and relatively benign. PSVT, by definition, is paroxysmas and, therefore, not sustained. PVCs can be a common occurrence in healthy individuals. Having a run of PVCs may be seen following cardiac injury. However, PVCs are individual beats and therefore not sustained.

A–389

(D) Propafenone has some beta adrenergic receptor blocking properties and may worsen heart failure. Amiodarone has demonstrated improvement in functional capacity in patients with heart failure. Dofetilide has a neutral effect on heart failure in the setting of atrial fibrillation. Digoxin was used for years in treating heart failure and would not be contraindicated in a person with both heart failure and atrial fibrillation.

Questions

Cardiovascular/Pharmacology

The acute treatment for deep venous thrombosis (DVT) is

(A) enoxaparin
(B) warfarin
(C) aspirin
(D) clopidogrel

Your Answer _____

_____

Cardiovascular

This condition, called "holiday heart syndrome," is sometimes associated with binge drinking. As many as 65% of all dysrhythmias found in persons under the age of 65 are a variation of "holiday heart syndrome." The dysrhythmia consists of

(A) frequent premature ventricular contractions
(B) paroxysmal atrial tachycardia
(C) atrial fibrillation
(D) type II A–V block

Your Answer _____

_____

Correct Answers

A–390

(A) The acute management of DVT consists of wearing compression stockings, elevating the leg, and administering anticoagulants. Enoxaparin is started first because it has an immediate onset of action. Long-term management involves administration of warfarin. Aspirin and clopidogrel inhibit platelet aggregation and are used preventively to inhibit blood clots in coronary artery disease, peripheral vascular disease, and cerebrovascular disease.

A–391

(C) The dysrhythmia associated with "holiday heart syndrome" is atrial fibrillation which can be very serious and the person should seek medical attention. If not life threatening, it usually resolves within 24 hours.

Questions

Gastroenterology/Surgery

Intussusception is a process in which a segment of intestine invaginates into the adjoining intestinal lumen, causing bowel obstruction. Surgery is definitive treatment, but which of the following may be tried prior to surgery if the patient has neither perforation nor peritonitis?

(A) Make the patient NPO to rest the bowel
(B) Administer metaclopramide
(C) Administer therapeutic enemas
(D) Administer analgesics

Your Answer _____

_____

Gastrointestinal/Surgery/Pediatrics

A mother brings her three-week-old baby boy in for evaluation of vomiting. The mother describes the vomiting as forceful and not just "spitting up" of formula. Palpation of the baby's abdomen reveals the presence of an olive-sized mass in the epigastrium. The diagnosis is

(A) pyloric stenosis
(B) intussusceptions
(C) lactose intolerance
(D) hiatal hernia

Your Answer _____

_____

Correct Answers

A–392

(C) Therapeutic enemas can be hydrostatic, with either barium or water-soluble contrast, or pneumatic, with air insufflations. The success rates vary from < 40% to > 90%. Analgesics could be administered to make the patient more comfortable but should not delay definitive treatment as bowel obstruction is a very serious condition. Resting the bowel and administration of metaclopramide has no merit in this condition.

A–393

(A) Pyloric stenosis is a condition that causes severe vomiting in the first few months of life. The pyloric muscle hypertropy results in narrowing of the pyloric canal which can become easily obstructed. Intussusception is marked by extreme abdominal pain due to invagination of one segment of the intestine into the adjoining intestinal lumen. Lactose intolerance means that the person cannot digest foods with lactose in them. A hiatal hernia is a condition in which part of the stomach protrudes upward through the opening at the esophagus and the diaphragm. It is characterized by "heartburn" and is not a surgical emergency.

Questions

Endocrinology

Your patient is confused about how to control her diabetes. She has been having normal blood sugars at bedtime but, upon awakening, she is hyperglycemic. She is not eating prior to bedtime and does not drink sugary drinks during the night. You believe she is experiencing the Somogyi effect. To verify this suspicion, you instruct the patient to

(A) decrease her 6 P.M. insulin dosage
(B) administer the long-acting insulin only in the morning
(C) check blood sugar nightly between 2–3 A.M.
(D) administer a low dose of regular insulin at bedtime

Your Answer _____

Women's Health

Preeclampsia is a condition in which hypertension arises during pregnancy. It is associated with protein in the urine. It often develops into eclampsia. What condition must be present to make the diagnosis of eclampsia?

(A) Proteinuria
(B) Peripheral and facial edema
(C) Tonic-clonic seizures
(D) Premature rupture of membranes

Your Answer _____

Correct Answers

A–394

(C) The Somogyi effect is also known as "rebound hyperglycemia" and is manifested as hypoglycemia followed by rebound hyperglycemia. To verify this phenomenon, the patient should check her blood sugar nightly between 2–3 A.M. One way to treat this phenomenon is to have a light bedtime snack, preferably protein. The other treatments mentioned do not apply to correction of this effect.

A–395

(C) Eclampsia is an acute and life-threatening complication of pregnancy and is characterized by the appearance of tonic-clonic seizures in a patient who had developed preeclampsia. Proteinuria and edema are manifestations of preeclampsia. Premature rupture of membranes refers to a patient who is beyond 37 weeks gestation and presents with rupture of membranes prior to onset of labor. It is not associated with preeclampsia.

Questions

Neurology/Pharmacology/Pediatrics

A mother brings in her seven-year-old daughter because she is concerned about a note sent from the child's teacher. The note says, "Julie is not paying attention, she often stares into space, blinking her eyes, and won't answer when I try to get her attention. She does this for only a few seconds and then she pays attention again. She is not disruptive, but the child is obviously distracted." The mother is seeking help because her daughter has always been a "model child." What medication will you prescribe?

(A) Methylphenidate
(B) Fluoxetine
(C) Alprazolam
(D) Ethosuximide

Your Answer _____

_____

Correct Answers

A–396

(D) This note from the teacher describes the child as having absence seizures. Ethosuximide is the drug of choice for children who have this type of seizure disorder. Methylphenidate is used in treating hyperactivity disorder, which this child does not have. Fluoxetine is an antidepressant and alprazolam is an antianxiety agent.

Questions

EENT

A 19-year-old college student presents with severe nasal congestion. He has suffered from seasonal allergies all his life but lately seems to be able to breathe only through his mouth. While talking to you, he uses a nasal spray containing phenylephrine to open his nostrils. Your physical examination is noncontributory except for the appearance of pale nasal mucosa bilaterally. This patient has

(A) allergic rhinitis
(B) rhinitis medicamentosa
(C) nasal polyps
(D) gustatory rhinitis

Your Answer _____

_____

Surgery/Emergency Medicine

Closing a wound too soon may increase infection risk in certain situations. In some cases, primary closure is contraindicated. Which one of the following should be delayed?

(A) Puncture wounds
(B) Animal bites to hands or feet
(C) Dirty wounds that are more than eight hours old
(D) All of the above require delayed closure.

Your Answer _____

_____

Correct Answers

A–397

(B) Many patients with a history of allergy and "stuffy nose" become addicted to nasal decongestants, a condition known as rhinitis medicamentosa. Allergic rhinitis may be seasonal, perennial, or occupational and the congestion will respond to nasal decongestants, which should only be used on a short-term basis to prevent the rebound congestion. Nasal polyps are growths inside the sinuses and nasal passages that can occur with allergic rhinitis, but these were not evident on the physical examination. Gustatory rhinitis is usually related to food or alcohol intake. People suffering from this form of rhinitis experience a clear, watery discharge, particularly after eating hot or spicy foods.

A–398

(D) All of the wounds are at increased risk of infection and closure should be delayed. When closure is delayed, the wound is still anesthetized, explored, cleaned, and debrided. It is then packed open and rechecked in 36 to 48 hours and again in 3 to 5 days. If the wound does not appear infected at the time of the second check, it can then be sutured.

Questions

Infectious Disease

Which drug, when combined with highly active antiretro-viral therapy (HAART), has been shown to flush HIV out of latent reservoirs?

(A) Fusion inhibitors
(B) Nicotinic acid (Niacin)
(C) Valproic acid
(D) Interferon

Your Answer _____

_____

Pulmonary

You are counseling a patient on smoking cessation. You tell her all of the following EXCEPT

(A) Smoking increases her risk for osteoporosis.
(B) One year after smoking cessation, her risk for a heart attack drops significantly.
(C) Cravings for nicotine after smoking cessation peaks at 3 days, diminishes over the following 3 to 4 weeks, and vanishes completely after six months.
(D) Smoking cessation at any age is associated with a decreased mortality rate.

Your Answer _____

_____

Correct Answers

A–399

(C) Valproic acid, a drug approved to treat bipolar disorder and epilepsy, has demonstrated an ability to stimulate the release of HIV from resting, infected T-cells. It is an inhibitor of a cellular enzyme crucial for keeping HIV genes hidden within the host cell's DNA. Only a few patients have received this treatment and the results show a decline in resting, infected cell numbers. Whether further investigation will prove beneficial overall remains to be seen.

A–400

(C) Nicotine withdrawal symptoms peak at 3 days and diminish over 3 to 4 weeks, but cravings for nicotine may last a lifetime. The remaining facts are all true.

Index

[Note: Numbers in the Index refer to question numbers.]

Notes

Notes

Notes

- Prednisone causes leukocytosis
- Ichthyosis = severe, persistent problems w/ dry skin
- Kalonychia = thin, concave nails w/ horizontal ridges often result from iron deficiency anemia.
- achalasia - birds beak

- "backwash iliatis" - Ulcerative colitis

- MC cause anal pain = anal fissure

- Methotrexate not useful for UC
- lordotic view is used to look @ lung apices

- ↑ TSH can be sign of acute HIV
- ↑ plt can be acute phase reactant